Experimental and Clinical
Pharmacology
with Special Topics

Experimental and Clinical
Pharmacology
with Special Topics

Vaishali Thakare
MBBS, MD (Pharmacology)
Assistant Professor, Department of Pharmacology
Dr DY Patil School of Medicine, Nerul, Navi Mumbai

Lily Dubey
MBBS, MD (Pharmacology)
Assistant Professor, Department of Pharmacology
Bundelkhand Medical College
Sagar, Madhya Pradesh

Kavitha Vivek Dongerkery
MBBS, MD (Pharmacology)
Assistant Professor, Department of Pharmacology
Dr DY Patil School of Medicine, Nerul, Navi Mumbai

Pramila Yadav
MBBS, MD (Pharmacology)
Professor, Department of Pharmacology
Dr DY Patil School of Medicine, Nerul, Navi Mumbai

CBS

CBS Publishers & Distributors Pvt Ltd
New Delhi • Bengaluru • Chennai • Kochi • Kolkata • Mumbai
Hyderabad • Jharkhand • Nagpur • Patna • Pune • Uttarakhand

Experimental and Clinical Pharmacology
with Special Topics

ISBN: 978-93-88108-46-1

Copyright © Authors and Publisher

First Edition: 2019
Reprint 2021

Published by Satish Kumar Jain and produced by Varun Jain for
CBS Publishers & Distributors Pvt Ltd
4819/XI Prahlad Street, 24 Ansari Road, Daryaganj, New Delhi 110 002, India
Ph: 011-23289259, 23266861, 23266867   Fax: 011-23243014
Website: www.cbspd.com   e-mail: delhi@cbspd.com; cbspubs@airtelmail.in

Corporate Office: 204 FIE, Industrial Area, Patparganj, Delhi 110 092, India
Ph: 011-49344934   Fax: 011-49344935   e-mail: publishing@cbspd.com; publicity@cbspd.com

Branches

• **Bengaluru:** Seema House 2975, 17th Cross, K.R. Road, Banasankari 2nd Stage, Bengaluru 560 070, Karnataka, India
  Ph: +91-80-26771678/79   Fax: +91-80-26771680   e-mail: bangalore@cbspd.com
• **Chennai:** 7, Subbaraya Street, Shenoy Nagar, Chennai 600 030, Tamil Nadu, India
  Ph: +91-44-26680620, 26681266   Fax: +91-44-42032115   e-mail: chennai@cbspd.com
• **Kochi:** 42/1325, 1326, Power House Road, Opposite KSEB, Power House, Ernakulum-682018, Kochi, Kerala, India
  Ph: +91-484-4059061-67   Fax: +91-484-4059065   e-mail: kochi@cbspd.com
• **Kolkata:** 6/B, Ground Floor, Rameswar Shaw Road, Kolkata-700 014 (WB), India
  Ph: +91-33-22891126, 22891127, 22891128   e-mail: kolkata@cbspd.com
• **Mumbai:** PWD Shed, Gala No. 25/26, Ramchandra Bhatt Marg, Next JJ Hospital Gate No. 2, Opp. Union Bank of India, Noorbaug, Mumbai-400009, Maharashtra, India
  Ph: +91-22-66661880/89   e-mail: mumbai@cbspd.com

Representatives

• **Hyderabad** 0-9885175004 • **Jharkhand** 0-9811541605 • **Nagpur**   0-9421945513
• **Patna**   0-9334159340 • **Pune**   0-9623451994 • **Uttarakhand** 0-9716462459

Printed at: Mudrak, Noida, UP, India.

to

---

my parents
late Mr Yadavrao and Mrs Satvsheela Deshmukh
and
my son Prasad & my husband Shirish

Preface

There are a lot of excellent books on pharmacology for postgraduate students. Postgraduate students have to take support of multiple sources for various topics in their PG syllabus like clinical pharmacology, experimental pharmacology, biostatistics and special topics like chronopharmacology, therapeutic drug monitoring, geriatric and paediatric pharmacology, etc. Considering the difficulties and stress a postgraduate faces during residency, we have made an attempt to compile the majority of the topics under one roof.

Hope you will make the most of it.

Thanking and wishing you a good luck!

Vaishali Thakare
Lily Dubey
Kavitha Vivek Dongerkery
Pramila Yadav

Acknowledgements

We would sincerely like to thank our family members for their support and encouragement. We also like to thank Mr YN Arjuna, Senior Vice President, Publishing, Editorial and Publicity, CBS Publishers & Distributors. We would take this opportunity to thank our Dean, Dr Surekha Patil, DY Patil Medical College, Nerul, Navi Mumbai; and Dr Bharti Kulkarni, Professor and Head, Paediatric Surgery, without whom this journey would have been incomplete.

Vaishali Thakare
Lily Dubey
Kavitha Vivek Dongerkery
Pramila Yadav

Contents

Section C: Biostatistics

Section D: Special Topics

Section A

Experimental Pharmacology

Experimental Animals

MOUSE

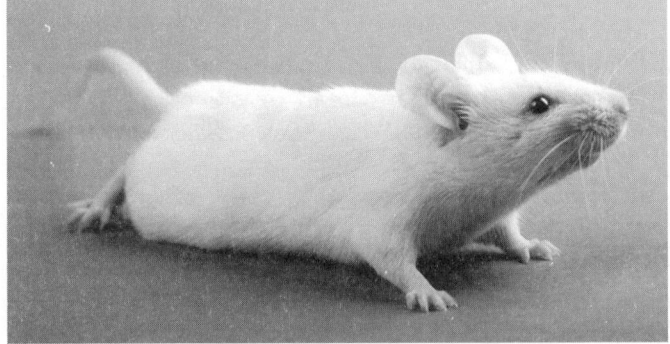

Fig. 1.1: Experimental animal—mouse

Important Points

Scientific name	*Mus musculus*
Average life span	1.5–2.5 years
Average weight (adult)	20–40 gm
Average age for experimentation (months)	0.75
Gestation period (days)	19–21 days
Daily food intake	4–5 gm
Heart rate and BP	780/min and 113/81 mmHg

Mice are the smallest rodents used in the biomedical research laboratory. They are very cheap, easy to maintain, handle, require small area for housing and very fast reproducibility. Most commonly used strains of mice are **Swiss albino** and **balb/c**.

Uses

- **Genetic studies:** Used widely in genetic studies because of their ability to add and selectively alter their genome (called transgenic animals). Examples of a few animal models for obesity and diabetes:
  - Yellow obese mouse
  - Obese mouse (ob/ob)
  - db/db
  - Japanese K/K
- Various human diseases like diabetes, atherosclerosis, endocrinal can be studied in detail by selective assessment at genetic level by *taking out selective gene (knockout)* and *insertion of selective gene (knock-in)*
- Acute toxicity study
- Screening of analgesics and chemotherapeutic agents
- Insulin assay
- Cancer research
- Evaluate drugs for teratogenicity

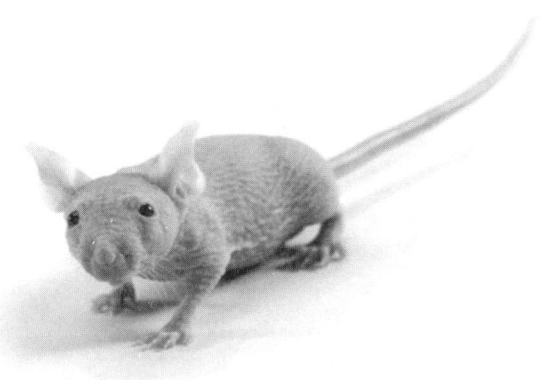

Fig. 1.2: Biege mouse—lack the NK cells and susceptible to cancer

Strains

1. **Nude mouse:**
   - Hairless genetic mutant
   - Lacks a thymus, deficient in T lymphocytes
   - Used in the research of transplantation and tissue immunity
   - Less susceptible to cancer and possess normal number of natural killer (NK) cells.

RAT

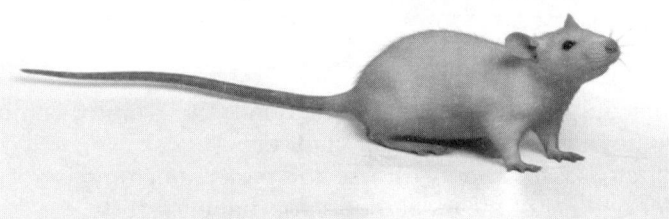

Fig. 1.3: Experimental animal—rat

Important Points

Scientific name	*Rattus norvegicus*
Average life span	2–3 years
Average weight (adult)	250 gm
Average age for experimentation (months)	1.5
Gestation period (days)	21–23 days
Daily food intake	10–20 gm
Heart rate and BP	300–500/min and 116/90 mmHg

Rat is commonly used in the experimental work because of its small size and greater sensitivity to most of the drugs. They are mostly preferred because of easy handling, sensitivity and low cost.

It is found to be very sturdy to withstand the long periods of experimentation under anaesthesia. Most standardized amongst all lab animals. It can be bred to obtain uniform and pure strain. Most popular strains of rat are Wistar rats and Sprague-Dawley rats. Important differences between the two strains are given below:

Wistar rat	Sprague-Dawley rat
Head is wide	Longer and narrower
Ears are long	Smaller ears
Tail length is shorter than the body length	Tail length is longer than the body length
Quiet and moderately prolific	Rapidly growing and prolific
Resistant to infection	Less resistant to infection, respiratory
Low incidence of tumours	Higher incidence

Anatomic Peculiarities

- Vomiting centre is absent in rat, hence they cannot vomit
- Do not have tonsil and gall bladder
- Pancreas is extremely diffuse and pancreatectomy is not easy. Hence it is not the ideal model for diabetes study.
- Stomach is divided in two parts by prominent white curved transverse ridge. Upper 2/5th is called rumen and lower 2/5th is called glandular secretory.
- Antifertility model. Estrous cycle is divided into four stages:
  - Oestrous
  - Met-oestrous
  - Dioestrous
  - Pro-oestrous

Uses

- Rats can be trained properly for various types of work performances, hence used in screening of **psychopharmacological agents**
- **Assay of different hormones**
- **Screening of antihypertensive drugs**
- **Cancer studies**
- Some of the popular genetic strains of rat develop for evaluation of obesity and diabetes mellitus—fatty (FA/FA) rat, hypertension—spontaneously hypertensive rat (SHR), salt-sensitive Dahl rat

Some important phenotypic differences between baby rats and mice
- Baby rat has blunt and broad large head relative to body, whereas mice have triangular, small head relative to body.
- Baby rat has small ears relative to the head, whereas mice have large ears.
- The baby rat hind paw and body ratio is larger as compared to mice.
- Tail is thick and shorter than body length in baby rat while mice have thin and larger or same length tail as compared to body.

GUINEA PIG

Important Points

Scientific name	Cavia Porcellus
Body weight	600–1200 gm
Life span	4–8 years
Food intake	6 gm/100 gm/day
Water intake	10 ml/100 gm/day
Gestation period	59–72 days
Heart rate and RR	230–380/min, 50–100/min

It is a very docile animal. Guinea pig (GP) is herbivorous and eats green foods, seeds and roots, but now in many laboratories feed is provided with a readymade chow diet which fulfils its daily dietary requirement. Guinea pigs are not able to synthesize the daily required vitamin C, hence it is essential to add vitamin C (ascorbic acid) in the chow. It is recommended that when GP is provided with the greens, then ascorbic acid should be given at the rate of 1 gm/L of drinking water on a weekly basis. If they are completely dependent on the chow, then vitamin C should be added in the dose of 200 mg/L daily.

Newborn GP can eat solid food by the fifth day and may be weaned by 2 weeks. Young GP are best mated after 3 months of age. The maturing is slow in male as compared with the female sibs. Coitus generally occurs at night and that followed by polygamous group mating. Duration of estrous cycle ranges from 13 to 20 days, an average of 16 days can be further divided into the other stages such as proestrus, metestrus and diestrus.

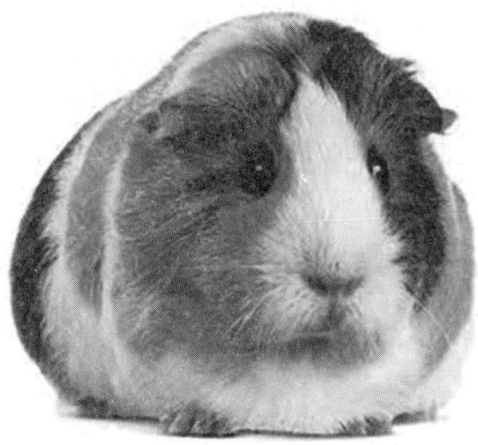

Fig. 1.4: Experimental animal—guinea pig

Uses

Evaluation model for
1. **Enteric amoebiasis:** Sensitive to various diseases and infections.
2. **Sensitisation studies:**
   • Highly sensitive to various antigens egg albumin.
   • Hypersensitivity and immune response, anaphylactic shock.
   • Encephalomyelitis, tuberculosis.
3. **Screening of bronchodilators**
   • Extremely sensitive to histamine.
   • Penicillin highly toxic—100–1000 times.
4. Study of local anaesthetics.
5. **Bioassay:** Digitalis, histamine and acetylcholine.
6. Guinea pig ileum is widely used for bioassay of histamine and acetylcholine.
7. **Special toxicity studies:** Dermal toxicity effect—skin is highly sensitive (GPM—guinea pig maximization test).
8. Screening of spasmodic and antispasmodic drugs.
9. **Hearing experiments:** Very sensitive cochlea.
10. **Study of ascorbic acid metabolism:** Guinea pig cannot synthesize vitamin C.

11. **L-asparaginase present in the serum:** Anti-leukemic property.

Guinea pig coronary arteries have duality concerning the origin and branching which are represented by 4 instead of 2 aortic branches compared to other species.

RABBIT—NON-RODENTS (MAMMALIANS)

General Information

Scientific name	Oryctolagus cuniculus
Body weight	1000–3500 gm
Life span	4–6 years
Gestational period	31 days
Food intake	5 gm/100 gm/day
Water	10 ml/100 gm/day
HR and BP	130–325/min, 90/60 mm Hg

The most common strain used is New Zealand white rabbit. Occurrence of atropinase (destroy atropine) makes it resistant to atropine.

Apart from the drugs, effects of skin creams, cosmetics, special diets, and food additives have also been tested on New Zealand white rabbits. Mainly, chemical method is preferred for **euthanasia** in rabbits. Cervical dislocation which is generally preferred for rodents is not suitable for rabbits because of short neck. Marginal ear vein is used for withdrawal of blood.

1. Standard animal for pyrogen testing of all solutions for human medical use.
2. To test toxic effects of cosmetics and pharmaceuticals.
3. Good model for the production of antibodies and antiserums.
4. Used in preclinical evaluation of different drugs for diseases like diabetes, diphtheria, tuberculosis, cancer, and heart diseases.
5. Screening of embryo toxic agents and teratogens.
6. **Historically used for pregnancy testing:** Injecting the serum from the patient into the rabbit and thereby inducing ovulation in the doe.

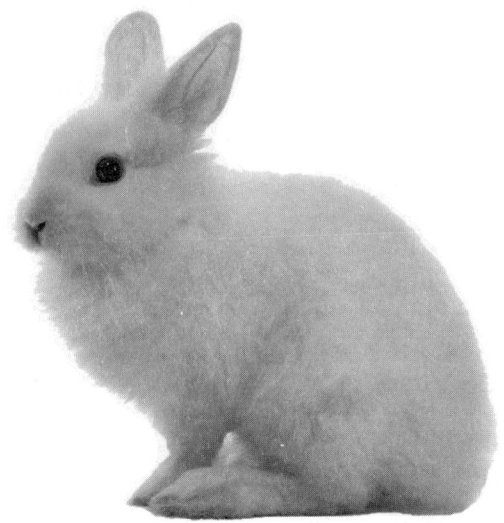

Fig. 1.5: Experimental animal—rabbit

7. **Biomedical research studies:** Genetics, nutrition, toxicology, physiology, immunology and reproduction.
8. **Reproduction research:** Non-spontaneous ovulation.
9. Commonly used to study the effect of drugs on pupil.
10. Animal of choice for many cardiac studies—because of its very simple cardiac conductive tissue.

DOG (CANIS FAMILIARIS)

Dog is the most preferred large experimental animal after monkey. The advantages being it has a small alimentary tract and can be trained easily. Most commonly used strains of dogs are Mongrel and Beagles. They are preferred for the experimental purposes due to manageable size, moderate length of hair coat, docile nature and ease to handle. Classical work of Pavlov's on conditioned reflexes was on dog.

Uses

1. Cardiovascular research is preferred in the dogs. Drugs acting on blood pressure and vascular system are preferably screened.

2. It is also a good model for diabetes mellitus and repro-duction—can develop spontaneous diabetes as in man.
3. Many human conditions in areas such as ulcerative colitis, open heart surgery, organ transplantation, central nervous system (CNS), safety pharmacology and toxicology.
4. Drugs for peptic ulcer screening.

BIBLIOGRAPHY

1. Falconer, DS (1976) in the UFAW handbook on the care and management of laboratory animals, 5th edition. (UFAW, Ed.) P.7, Churchill Livingstone, Edinburgh
2. Guide for care and use of laboratory animal–Institute of Laboratory Animal Resources Commission on Life Sciences—National Research Council.
3. Jackson F, Scott PP. Laboratory animal 1970;4:135–137.
4. Medhi B, Prakash A. Practical manual of clinical and experimental Pharmacology, New Delhi, Jaypee Brothers Medical Publication, Second edition, 2017.

Effect of Drugs on Dog: Blood Pressure and Respiration

PROCEDURE

RECORDING OF THE BLOOD PRESSURE

ANIMAL

Dog (commonly used species of dog for the experiment is Mongrel) is obtained from a municipal pound. It is a stray animal, hence it needs to be kept for quarantine for period of 15 days (isolated to know the antimicrobial status). Before starting the procedure one has to tie the mouth of the dog to prevent biting and the animal should be weighed to calculate the drug doses.

Anaesthesia

Most preferred anaesthetic agent used is chloralose because it has the advantage of better cardiovascular and respiratory stability. Alternatively pentobarbitone, an intermediately acting barbiturate, can be used in the dose of 35 mg/kg/IP. It has rapid onset of action. Loss of corneal reflex is a guide to depth of anaesthesia. If necessary give intermittent doses to prolong the duration of action. It has vagolytic action and depresses autonomic ganglion. Anaesthetic is injected through the saphenous vein.

Femoral Vein Cannulation

Once the animal is anaesthetised cannulate the femoral vein for administration of drugs. Femoral vein is the bluish non-pulsatile structure lying below the superfacial fascia parallel to femoral artery. Isolate segment of vein by passing the twin ligature. After that arterial cannula is passed in femoral vein with the help of cannula director, then it is fixed by ligating distal thread in twin ligature. Three-way connection is fixed to the arterial cannula and flushed with normal saline.

Tracheal Cannulation

Next step is to expose the trachea and cannulate it. A midline incision is made on the skin of the neck starting from the lower end of larynx up to the upper end of thorax. Subcutaneous fat is cleared and para-tracheal muscles are separated to expose trachea with the help of a pair of scissors by introducing the closed tips and then separating the blades. A thick twin ligature is passed below the tracheal segment after lifting it with artery forceps. A transverse cut is made in between two rings so as to make an opening for the introduction of the tracheal cannula. The cannula is introduced into the opening pointing towards the lungs and held firmly in position with the help of a twin ligature.

Tracheal cannula is introduced for the following purposes:
1. Increased trachea-bronchial secretions under anaesthesia is removed out by using suction cannula and to allow free breathing without any obstruction.
2. We can connect the tracheostomy tube to the machine called Mary's tambour so that respiratory movement can be noted.
3. To provide artificial respiration with the help of a respiratory pump when required. The volume of air per stroke of the pump and the rate are adjusted depending on the species of the animal.

Isolation of Carotid Artery and its Cannulation

Next step is to cannulate carotid artery for recording of blood pressure. Carotid artery runs parallel and close to the trachea on either side along with the internal jugular veins and vago-sympathetic trunk and easily recognized by their elastic and pulsating nature. One of these arteries is cleaned from the accompanying structures for a sufficient length with the help of a blunt dissector. It is then tied as near the head end as possible, a bulldog clamp is placed about 3 cm nearer the heart and a thread is passed round the artery. A cut is made carefully on the artery close to the first ligature with the help of a sharp curved scissors so as to make a small opening through which an arterial cannula is connected to the rubber tubing which is connected to mercury manometer. This mercury manometer is connected to Mariotte's bottle which contains anticoagulant (sodium citrate) solution. Complete system is filled with an anticoagulant solution to remove the air bubbles. The three-way tap in the manometer is then turned so as to fill one limb, the connecting tubings and the cannula with the anticoagulant fluid from the reservoir bottle. The pinch-cock on the short tubing attached to the side tube of the artery cannula is opened at the same time so as to allow the coagulant fluid to run out. When the whole system is rendered free of air bubbles, the pinch-cock is closed again. The pressure in the manometer is then increased to about 150 mmHg and the three-way tap turned so that the manometer now remains in communication only with the cannula. The positive pressure, being approximately equal to that of the blood in the animal, prevents too much blood from coming out of the animal's artery into the recording system. Before the bulldog clamp is removed, 0.5 ml of 1% heparin solution is injected into the arterial cannula through the rubber tubing, the bulldog clamp is then taken off; the column of mercury rises or falls slightly until its pressure counterbalances that of the blood. The writing point remains at a constant level except for slight oscillations due to the heart beats and the respiratory movements. The height of the mercury column midway between the top and bottom of these oscillations is taken as the mean arterial pressure. The femoral vein is exposed by a midline incision on the medial surface of the upper part of the thigh. In rabbit, usually the external jugular vein is exposed just under the skin at the side of the neck taking special care because of its fragility. The venous cannula is inserted into the vein in the same fashion as into the artery except that the bulldog clamp is first applied proximally and a ligature tied a little distally while the vein is full with blood. After the cannula is tied in position it is connected with a burette filled with warm saline. Drugs are injected through the rubber tubing close to the cannula and a constant volume of saline is allowed to run each time after injection.

Normal variations in the blood pressure is recorded. A steadily rising baseline, when the blood in the arterial cannula appears dark, suggests anoxia. Occasionally, after switching to artificial respiration a spiky base line may occur. This is often an indication that the animal is trying to breathe against the artificial respiration. An erratic baseline also occurs when the anaesthesia is too light or the bladder is full. The tracings of the normal blood pressure record show that in addition to the variations in pulse pressure (**waves of the first order** due to heart beats), there are sometimes variations with respiration (**waves of the second order**). The blood pressure somewhat rises with each inspiration and drops with each expiration due to an increased blood flow to the heart during inspiration, concomitant acceleration of heart, and spread of the stimulation from the respiratory to the vasomotor centres producing slight vasoconstriction.

Respiration Recording

Very large respiratory waves (Traube-Hering curves) are sometimes observed during abnormally slow respiration caused by 'explosions' of the strong excitation in the respiratory centre. The blood pressure curve sometimes shows slow waves each taking in a period of eight or more respiratory movements (waves of the third order or Meyer's waves). They are dependent on changes in nervous control of blood vessels, and arise when insufficient blood flows to the cerebrum, or during increase in intracranial pressure. These are also commonly seen after haemorrhage due to the following mechanism. As the blood pressure falls due to haemorrhage, chemoreceptor stimulation occurs due to stagnant anoxia of the chemoreceptor glomus tissue resulting in reflex vasoconstriction. The systemic pressure there upon rises, and as a result, the chemoreceptor stimulation dies away as the blood flow to the glomus cells improves. This results in a reduction in reflex vasoconstriction, producing a fall in blood pressure once again, thus repeating the cycle. These Meyer's waves are always accentuated by bilateral carotid occlusions and are abolished by cutting the chemoreceptor nerves.

Adrenergic Receptor and their Sites

β_1: Sites are myocardium and JG cells of kidney—↑ in blood pressure

β_2: Skeletal muscle vasculature — ↓ in blood pressure

β_3: Adipose tissue

α_1: Blood vessels of skin and mucus membrane—marked ↑ in blood pressure

α_2: Presynaptically

Characteristics of β receptors

• Highly sensitive, hence get activated at low dose and long-lasting response.

• Response of these receptors is masked by α-receptor response.

α-Receptors

Predominant in numbers, require higher concentration and short lasting.

Effect of Adrenaline on Blood Pressure

Explanation: Adrenaline acts on β_1, β_2 and α_1.

In low dose: Only β_2 receptors get activated, hence only fall in BP is seen.

In moderate dose: Initial marked rise in blood pressure because of activation of α_1 and β_1 receptors followed by slight fall because of β_2 response which is long lasting.

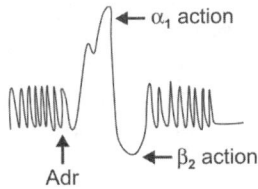

Fig. 2.1: Effect of adrenaline on blood pressure

Noradrenaline: Only sharp rise in blood pressure but fall is not seen because of no β_2 action of NA.

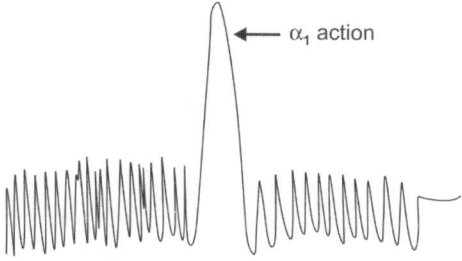

Fig. 2.2: Effect of noradrenaline on BP

Isoprenaline: Initial slight rise (β_1) followed by sustained fall (β_2) is seen as isoprenaline is predominant β_2 agonist.

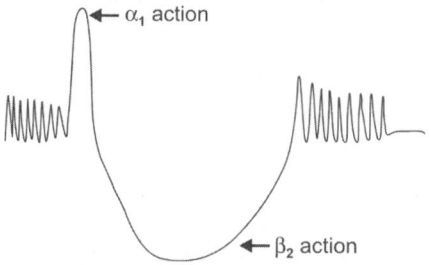

Fig. 2.3: Effect of isoprenaline on BP

Histamine: Fall in blood pressure because of stimulation of H_1 receptor on vascular smooth muscle.

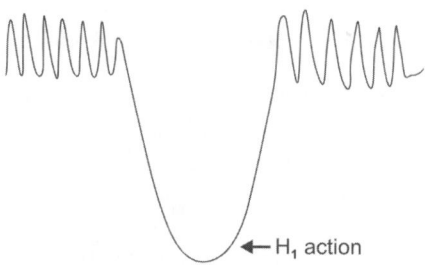

Fig. 2.4: Effect of histamine on BP

Acetylcholine: Sharp and short-lasting fall in blood pressure (M_3) receptor action. It is degraded by acetylcholinesterase enzyme.

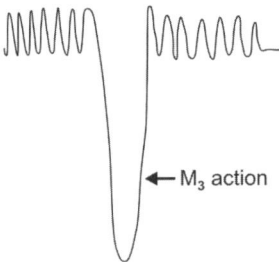

Fig. 2.5: Effect of acetylcholine on BP

EFFECT ON RESPIRATION

Adrenaline: Increase amplitude and transient apnoea. Increase amplitude is β_2 action. Transient apnoea is because of reflex respiratory centre inhibition.

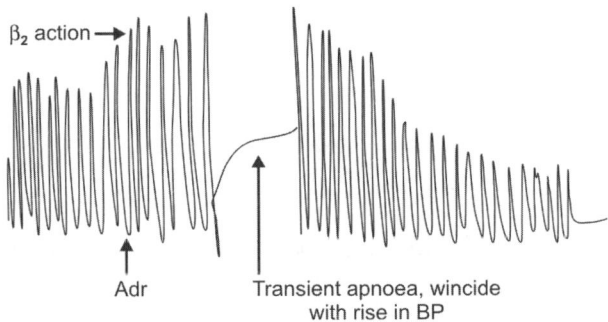

Fig. 2.6: Effect of adrenaline on respiration

Noradrenaline: Transient apnoea but no change in amplitude as NA does not have β_2 action. Transient apnoea is because of reflex respiratory centre inhibition.

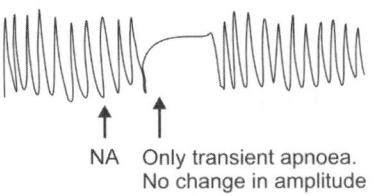

Fig. 2.7: Effect of noradrenaline on respiration

Isoprenaline: Predominant β_2 action, hence shows increase amplitude of respiration (β_2).

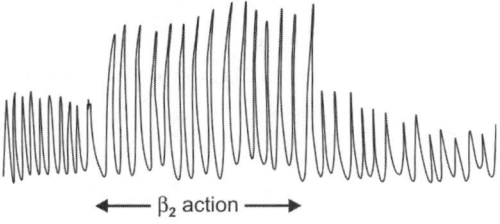

Fig. 2.8: Effect of isoprenaline on respiration

Histamine: Reduce amplitude because of bronchospasm due to H_1 mediated response.

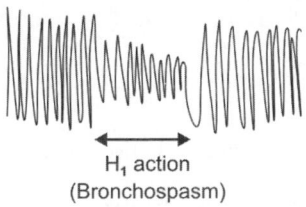

Fig. 2.9: Effect of histamine on respiration

Acetylcholine: Reduced amplitude because of broncho-spasm. This effect is due to M_3 receptor in the bronchial smooth muscles.

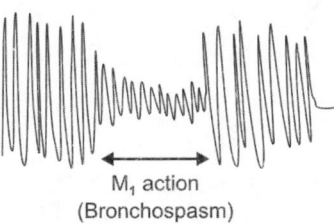

Fig. 2.10: Effect of acetylcholine on respiration

Autonomic Phenomenon

1. Potentiation

Pressor: Adrenaline is administered and there is rise in blood pressure. Once the blood pressure touches the baseline ephedrine is administered and it shows rise in blood pressure. Adrenaline is repeated in the same dose after ephedrine and it shows rise in blood pressure which is more than the previous. This potentiation is because ephedrine has inhibited the reuptake of adrenaline. Ephedrine is indirectly acting sympathomimetic, hence facilitate the release of adrenaline at postganglionic sympathetic nerve endings.

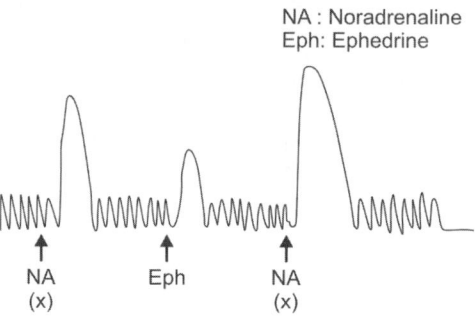

NA : Noradrenaline
Eph: Ephedrine

NA
(x)   Eph   NA
              (x)

Fig. 2.11: Pressor action of adrenaline

Depressor: Effect of acetylcholine on blood pressure is facilitated by physostigmine. Physostigmine is a reversible anticholinesterase and prevents the degradation of acetylcholine.

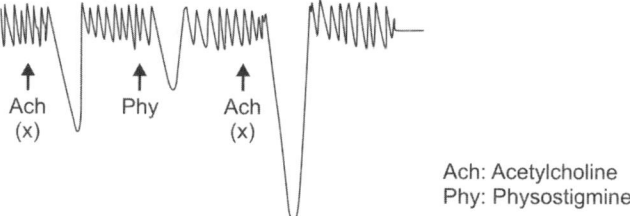

Ach
(x)   Phy   Ach
              (x)

Ach: Acetylcholine
Phy: Physostigmine

Fig. 2.12: Depressor action of acetylcholine on blood pressure

2. Tachyphylaxis (Acute Tolerance)

When tyramine is administered frequently at short interval in same doses the pharmacological response reduces. This phenomenon is called tachyphylaxis. Tyramine is indirectly acting sympathomimetics. When administered at short interval it depletes the stores of catecholamine at postganglionic sympathetic nerve endings.

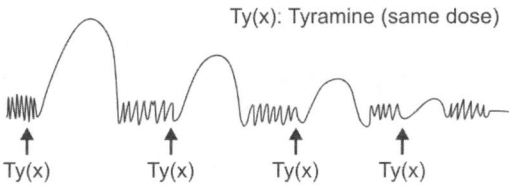

Fig. 2.13: Tyramine-induced acute tolerance

3. Dales Vasomotor Reversal

Sir Dales has first demonstrated this phenomenon. There is rapid rise in blood pressure (α_1) when adrenaline is given intravenously followed by fall (β_2). When α-blocker is administered after adrenaline, there is only fall because α_1 action is blocked. This phenomenon is not seen with noradrenaline.

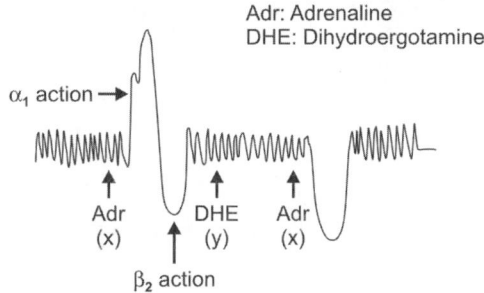

Fig. 2.14: Dales vasomotor reversal phenomenon

4. Nicotinic Action of Acetylcholine

Acetylcholine in smaller doses shows fall in blood pressure (M_3). Atropine is given to block the action, muscarinic action of acetylcholine. Acetylcholine is repeated to check the

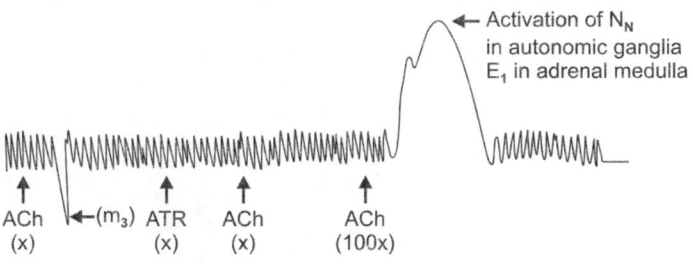

Fig. 2.15: Nicotinic action of acetylcholine

competency of block. Later on acetylcholine is repeated in very doses to activate nicotinic receptors situated in autonomic ganglion and adrenal medulla. There is M shape rise in blood pressure because of profound release of catecholamine in circulation.

BIBLIOGRAPHY

1. Ghosh MN, Fundamentals of Experimental Pharmacology, Kolkata Scientific Book Agency, 3rd edition, 2017.
2. Thakare V. and Yadav P, Practical Manual of Dental Pharmacology and Viva Voce, Experimental Pharmacology, Page no 18–36, Mumbai Bhalani Publishing House, 2018.

Anaesthesia in Experimental Animals

In biomedical research animal experiment is done with conscious animal only when it is not possible to study in anaesthetized animal.

AIM OF THE ANAESTHESIA

- To provide analgesia, amnesia and immobilization of animal.
- To exclude stress and discomfort which can affect the pharmacological effect and reproducibility of data.

Care to be Taken

During anaesthesia one should take care of circulation and oxygenation.

Methods of Anaesthesia

Animal can be anaesthesised by:

Local anaesthesia: Only the selected part of the body is anaesthetized.

It is less commonly preferred (calm animals like sheep). In this technique animal remains conscious. This can be induced by simple application of the local anaesthetic solution (surface anaesthesia).

Local anaesthetic solution can be injected in the skin/subcutaneous tissue.

Most commonly used drugs are: Lignocaine, bupivacaine.

Advantages: No special arrangement is required. It does not affect the physiological functions of animal.

Disadvantages: Require skilled person for administration. Onset time is 15 minutes and last for 45 minutes.

General anaesthesia: In this type animal is made unconscious.

General condition of animal including renal, hepatic, cardiac and pulmonary function has to be assessed.

This can be induced by inhalational or injectable route.

Inhalational: Volatile gases like halothane, isoflurane, enflurane are used. Ether has disadvantage of high inflammability, still it was used till recently. Inhalational mixture should include 21% of oxygen. N_2O can be added with O_2 and inhalational agent. this reduces the requirement of agent. This technique requires special instrument like vaporizer. It is short lasting. It has minor role in small animals and used for larger animals.

INTRAVENOUS AGENTS

Barbiturates

In this group agents like pentobarbitone and thiopentone are used. Pentobarbitone is short and rapid acting. It has vagolytic effect, hence it is not used for CVS drugs. Thiopentone is ultrashort acting.

Chloralose

Compound of chloral and glucose. Alpha chloralose is the active form. Soluble in hot water, alcohol and ether. It is prepared as 1% solution and administered IV or intraperitoneal. Preferred for rapid onset and irreversible anaesthesia in dog and cat.

Advantages

• Uniform depth
• No effect on respiration and circulation
• ANS—reflexes not depressed.

Urethane

Water soluble and use in 25% concentration. It is preferred for short-term experiments. As it has hepatotoxic effect, it also causes agranulocytosis and pulmonary adenoma. It has slight depressive effect on ANS reflexes, hence not preferred for CVS studies.

Paraldehyde

Wide safety margin. It has slight depressive effect on ANS reflexes, hence not preferred for CVS studies.

BIBLIOGRAPHY

1. NS Parmar, Shiv Prakash, Screening methods in Pharmacology, New Delhi, Narosa Publishing House.

Euthanasia Methods in Experimental Animals

Euthanasia means the humane killing/sacrifice of an animal which produces rapid unconsciousness and subsequent death without or minimal pain or distress to animal.

The experimental animals have to be sacrificed for different reasons as outlined below:

1. *Experiments on isolated tissues (in vitro):* Requires biological materials, e.g. isolated smooth muscles, heart, nerve-muscle preparations, etc.
2. Application of irreversible general anaesthesia.
3. Irreversible damage, pain, distress and suffering more than acceptable limits or may persist for a long time after the completion of experiments.

There are various methods available for euthanasia. The choice of a method depends on species, age, and availability of restraint and skill of the individuals performing euthanasia.

The method used for euthanasia must be:

- Reliable and should be irreversible.
- It should cause minimum pain, distress, anxiety or apprehension.
- It should cause rapid loss of consciousness.
- It should be safe for the scientist, should not cause emotional effect on personnel.
- Animal should not be sacrificed in a room where other animals (same species) are being housed.

The methods of euthanasia in experimental animals are divided in two broad categories:

1. Physical method 2. Chemical method

1. Physical Method

Trained and experienced personnel and functioning equipment is important for this.

Various techniques are:

- **Cervical dislocation:** This is frequently used for small animals weighing less than 1 kg, e.g. mice, rats, guinea pig, rabbits and other rodents.
- **Decapitation:** Instrument called guillotine is generally used. This method is commonly used for rodents and small rabbits.
- **Exanguination:** Bleeding till death. Practiced in small animals like rat and hamster.

2. Chemical Methods

Anaesthetics in overdose cause rapid unconsciousness which is followed by death. Inhalational and Intravenous anaesthetics are used.

Inhalational anaesthetics: Volatile anaesthetics at a high concentration of 80–100% produce unconsciousness and death. Agents like halothane, enflurane, sevoflurane, methoxyflurane, isolfulrane and desflurane are preferred for euthanasia in animals.

Carbon dioxide (CO_2): This method is widely used and effective also. It causes rapid hypoxia followed by depression of vital centres. It is used as 20–70% of the chamber volume per minute. This method is preferred in several animal but it is dangerous to use, hence needs to take precaution.

Carban monoxide
Carbon dioxide (CO_2) + chloroform
Halothane

INTRAVENOUS ANAESTHETICS

1. **Sodium-pentobarbitone:** This is intermediate acting barbiturate. Rapid loss of consciousness, hence very effective and method of first choice for producing euthanasia. Dose for euthanasia is very high and almost three times the anaesthetic dose. Route can be intravenous in larger animals (nonrodents). It can be given by intraperitoneal route in small animals.

2. **Chloral hydrate:** Not recommended in small animals. Only recommended in larger animals by IV route.

3. **Ketamine:** Given by IM route. Acceptable for both small and large animals.

METHODS NOT ACCEPTABLE BY CPCSEA GUIDELINES

Physical—decompression, stunning, electrocusion

Chemical—nitrogen, argon, curare like drugs (muscle relaxants), nicotine, $MgSO_4$, KCl, strychnine, paraquate, air embolism.

BIBLIOGRAPHY

1. Guidelines on the regulation of Scientific experiments on animals, Ministry of Environment and Forest (Animal Welfare Division), Govt. of India, June 2007.
2. Miller EV, Ben M, Cass JS, Comparative anaesthesia in Laboratory animals. Fedproc 1969; 28:1369–1586.

5

Blood Collection in Experimental Animals

PURPOSE OF BLOOD COLLECTION

Blood collection is done in experimental animals for various purposes like:

1. To study effect of drug on hematological and biochemical parameters
2. To study pharmacokinetic parameters of drugs like metabolism, elimination, etc.

There are various techniques for blood collection and broadly classified as:

- Terminal method
- Non-terminal methods
- Selection of method depends upon the factors like
  - Amount of blood required
  - Body weight of animal

Important factors should be considered while collecting blood

1. **Amount of blood to be collected:** Blood volume of animal varies with body weight. It is roughly 55–70 ml/kg. Approximately 10% of blood volume can be removed at once, withdrawl of >15% blood volume can affect adversely to the animal in the form of reduced RBC. It can also cause haemorrhagic shock and death. If it is multiple withdrawal, it should be 1% of blood volume, i.e. 0.6 ml.

2. **Site selection and dilatation of vein:** One should remove the debris and hairs at the site. To make it prominent it has

to be dilated by dipping into warm water (45°C)/applying xylene (it is carcinogenic).
3. **Needle size:** It should be less than the diameter of vein. Length of the needle varies from 1 to 5 cm and diameter should be 17–27 G. It should cause minimum trauma.

Various Techniques for Blood Collection

Terminal	*Nonterminal*
• Animal is made unconscious by physical stunning and laparotomy done after decapitation.	• Restraint is the main disadvantage.
	• Mainly preferred in smaller animals.
	• Skilled persons are required and should be done under anaesthesia.
• Example: Blood is withdrawn from IVC/ aorta, cardiac puncture. In smaller animal retroorbital bleeding.	• Tip of tail, superficial veins, permanent venous cannulation, retro-orbital bleeding, smaller animals like mouse/rat preferred.
• Larger amount of blood is withdrawn.	• Can cause haematoma and blindness because of pressure on optic nerve

Procedure for Blood Collection

• **Step I**
  ⬩ Clean the site (hair) by clipping
  ⬩ Apply antiseptic solution
• **Step II**
  ⬩ Identify the vein
  ⬩ Dilate and fix it
• **Step III**
  ⬩ Pierce the skin and vein with 45° angle
  ⬩ Collect blood in heparinised container/vacutainer

BIBLIOGRAPHY

1. Besch EL, Chou BJ. Physiological responses to blood collection methods in Rats. Proceedings of the Society of Experimental Biology and Medicine 1971; 138:1019–21.
2. Ladwig J, Stribrny K. A simplified method for stress free continuous blood collection in large animals. Laboratory animal science 1988; 31:5–18.

6

Bioassay

ASSAY

Estimation of concentration of active principle in unit quantity of the given preparation.

Different Types of Assays

1. **Chemical assay:** Estimation of potency by chemical methods, e.g. spectrophotometry.
2. **Immunoassay:** Estimation of potency by immunological methods, e.g. radioimmunoassay.
3. **Bioassay:** Estimation of potency by biological means.

Definition of Bioassay

It is defined as estimation of relative potency of active principle in the test solution by comparing with standard solution on living tissue (intact animal/isolated tissue).

Bioassay was started in the late 18th century, when standardization of diphtheria antitoxin was done by **Paul Ehrlich.**

Principles of Bioassay

1. Biological response produced by the active principle (to be bio-assayed) has to be same in all animal species.
2. **Sensitivity:** Quantity of response produced by particular dose should be same in same animal when tested at different times or all animals of same species at same time, provided that the conditions are constant, e.g. degree of rise in BP by particular dose of adrenaline should be same.

3. Standard solution should have same activity as the test solution.
4. Activity assayed should be of interest.
5. **Specificity:** Same response can be obtained by two different drugs, e.g. histamine and acetylcholine will cause contraction of guinea pig ileum. Hence, for histamine bioassay muscarinic receptors should be blocked by atropine.
6. Method should be reproduced and stable over a period of time.
7. Individual variation should be considered and minimized.

Advantages of Bioassay

1. Highly sensitive, specific, reproducible, precision, accuracy, stability
2. Simple and fast procedure
3. Can be possible with less amount of test solution.

Disadvantages

1. Time consuming, cumbersome
2. Loss of tissue sensitivity over a period of time
3. *Errors:* Biological and methodological
4. Only toxicity and high dose study is possible, dose ranging study cannot be possible.

Indications/Applications/Uses

1. Active principle has some pharmacological action but chemical structure is not known, e.g. LATS—long acting thyroid stimulants.
2. When chemical assays are complicated/insensitive, e.g. adrenaline, histamine. By bioassay this can be measured in μgm.
3. Estimation of biological activity of substance which are obtained from natural source, e.g. penicillin G.
4. Evaluation/screening of new compound for biological activity, e.g. new drug development.
5. Study of LD 50/ED 50
6. Biological standardization of drugs from natural sources which cannot be obtained in pure form, e.g. oxytocin, heparin, insulin.

7. To compare the strength of an active compound obtained from various sources, e.g. cardiac glycosides.
8. Compound with similar structure but different biological activity, e.g. sufonamides and thiazides.
9. Commercial production of drugs like antibiotics.
10. Standardization of vaccines, biologics, antisera, disinfectants and antiseptics.

Examples of Certain Important Bioassays

Whole Animal Assays

- **Vasopressin:**
  - ◆ Anaesthetized rat rise in blood pressure.
  - ◆ Hydrated rat increase in urine output.
- **Estrogen:** Vaginal cornification seen in ovariectomised rat
- **Insulin:** Hypoglycemic convulsions in mice
- **D-Tc:** Head drop relaxation of neck muscles in rabbit
- **Cardiac glycoside:** Death of guinea pig

Isolated Tissue

- **Acetylcholine:** Dorsal muscle of leech, frog rectus abdominus, guinea pig tracheal chain, ascending and descending colon—rat
- **Histamine:** Guinea pig ileum
- **Adrenaline:** Rat uterus diestrus
- **Oxytocin:** Estogen primed uterus in rat
- **5-HT:** Gastric fundus

This can be further classified as:

- **Slow contracting:** Frog rectus abdominus muscle, stomach fundus, guinea pig tracheal smooth muscle, biventer cervicis muscle of chick.
- **Fast contracting:** Ileum, uterus, ascending and descending colon, etc.

CELL LINE

- Isolated Leydig cell line: *In vitro* testosterone synthesis—LH hormone.
- Highly advanced research
  Micro-organisms: Vitamin B_{12}—growth of euglena gracilis, tetracycline—bacillus pumilus.

Types of Bioassay

A. **Indirect:** Log dose response curve of test solution is compared with the LDR of standard and by comparison the potency is obtained, e.g. in estimation of potency of ergotamine in crude preparation, it is injected in white leg horn cock. This causes vasoconstriction and bluish dis colouration of the comb. The intensity of colour varies with the dose.

B. **Direct:** Threshold dose required for predetermined response is measured for direct and test solution directly. Relative potency of the test compound is obtained by taking the ratio between these doses, e.g. digitalis assay in cat.

Parameter evaluated—amount of solution required to stop the heart beat (cardiac arrest)

Threshold dose of standard = total period of infusion × rate of drug administration.

Concentration of test = threshold dose of standard/threshold dose of test × concentration of standard

Quantal Assay/Direct End Point Assays

In this method the dose of standard and test/unkown solution required to obtain the pre-determined "all or none" response measured. Then by comparing them the potency ratio is calculated.

Pre-determined "all or none" response: Some examples are:
- Digitalis induced cardiac arrest in guinea pig/cat
- Head drop assay for d-tubocurarine in rabbit
- Insulin induced hypoglycemic convulsions in mice.

Graded Response Assays

In this assay the response of varying doses (ascending order) of standard and test solution is measured on same tissue.

Examples: Bioassay of histamine on guinea pig ileum, bioassay of acetylcholine on frog rectus abdominis muscle.

Standardization

Same amount of response should be seen to the particular dose after repeat of same.

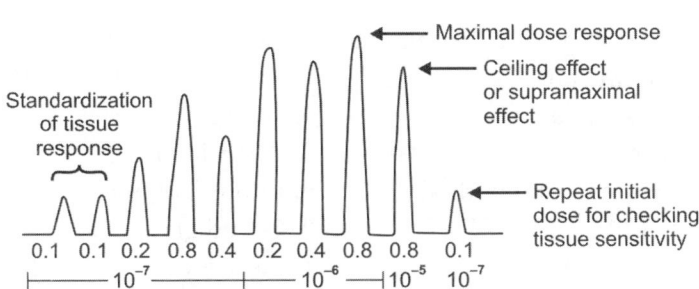

Fig. 6.1: Standardization of assembly

Errors in Bioassay

While performing bioassay, there may be variation seen in the response. It may be increased/decreased. This could be because of biological/methodological errors.

Biological Errors

This can be because of errors in:

1. **Animal selection/handling:**
   - Animal should be healthy, species, sex, age, weight should be considered.
   - Animal must be handled by qualified and trained staff and should be housed properly before experiment.
2. **Tissue handling**
   - Repeated washing can cause downregulation of receptors and reduction in response.
   - Over a period sensitivity of tissue may be lost—change the tissue.
   - Minimum handling and cleaning of the tissue while isolation and mounting in the organ bath.

Methodological Error

These errors are made by experimenter and commonly at following places:

- **Physiological salt solution (PSS) preparation:** Avoid vigorous mixing of ingredients
- While making serial dilution of the drug.
- During the response recording.

Various pieces of equipment required for bioassay:

1. Organ bath
2. Rotating drum
3. Kymograph
4. Tissue holder with air supply
5. Writing lever
6. Fulcrum
7. Stirrer
8. Perfusion bottle
9. Rubber tubing
10. Coiled glass tube
11. Electric supply

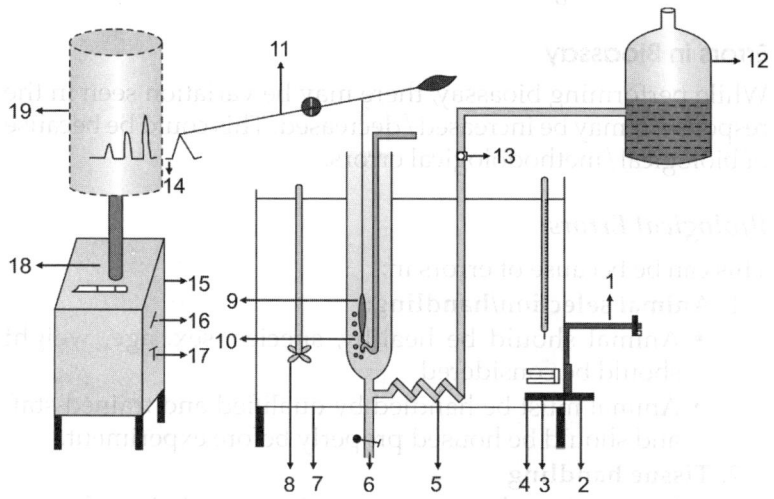

Fig. 6.2: Schematic diagram of organ bath set up for bioassay

Names

1. Power input
2. Switch board
3. Heating rod
4. Thermostat
5. Coiled glass tube
6. Inner bath outlet
7. Outer bath
8. Stirrer
9. Tissue
10. Airator
11. Lever
12. Mariotte's bottle
13. Clamp
14. Stylus
15. Electric motor
16. Gear
17. Clutch lever
18. Drum rotator indicator
19. Sherrington's rotating drum

ORGAN BATH

This was first discovered by Rudolph Magnus in 19th century for an experiment intestinal strips. It has two parts:

Internal organ bath for holding the tissue. Internal organ bath is a glass test tube with capacity of 5–50 ml. It has inlet connected with coiled glass tube and outlet for removal of PSS after wash.

Outer organ bath: It provides a water jacket to internal organ bath for maintaining the proper temperature. It is made up of steel/perspex glass/glass. Perspex is durable material. Required temperature is 37°C.

- **Single unit organ bath:** It has only one internal organ bath. Developed by Rudolph Magnus.
- **Double or multiple unit organ baths:** This was developed by Gaddum. It has double unit organ bath with two inner tissue organ bath.
- **Electric connection:** Outer organ bath has facility to connect with electric circuit.
- **Thermostat and heating coil:** Heating coil maintains the temperature outside the inner bath, also the PSS in the inner jacket and the coiled glass tube immersed in the outer jacket. Thermostat maintains static or constant temperature throughout the experiment and prevent the wide variation.
- **Stirrer:** To provide uniform temperature throughout the organ bath.
- **Fulcrum:** Writing lever is fixed to this which in turn is attached to the outer organ bath. It allows free movement of lever for recording of response on the drum.
- **Rotating drum and kymograph:** This is also called Sherrington's rotating drum. It has lever and gear for adjustment of speed. Speed varies with the contraction of tissue. For slow contracting tissue speed should be less and vice versa. Speed of the drum is 1 revolution per 96 min.
- **Kymograph:** The paper which is attached to the drum and the response is recorded on it. It has rough inner side which is in contact with the drum. Outer side is smooth and glossy which is easier for recording the graph.
- **Smoking of the drum:** The kymograph paper is wrapped smoothly around the drum and secured tightly with the

adhesive. Burning cotton soaked in benzene or kerosene is used for smoking. Drum has to be kept at sufficiently high distance to prevent fire. It is rotated with reasonable speed to obtain a thin and uniform smoking. Nowadays **inked-kymograph** is used.

• **Fixing of the graphs:** This is done with the help of fixing solution at the end of the experiment. Shellac and colophony is used to make the fixing solution.

Procedure for making the fixing solution: Powdered shellac is mixed in methyl alcohol and dissolved till it gets saturated and precipitated, then keep solution for 5–7 days so that the particles get settle down at the bottom. Decantation of the solution is done to get non-precipitated solution. Store the prepared fixing solution in the cool and dark place.

Perfusion bottle and rubber tubing: It contains the PSS and has outlet at the bottom which is connected to the rubber tubing which is connected to coiled glass tube.

Tissue holder and air supply: It is attached to the outer organ bath. Tissue is attached to it and it is present inside the internal organ bath. It also supplies the air/O_2 to the tissue and help in mixing the tyrode.

PHYSIOLOGICAL SALT SOLUTION (PSS)

Physiological salt solution is necessary to keep tissue viable outside the body. It provides ionic and nutritional supply to the tissue. There are different types of PSS and selection of them varies with the tissue. Distilled or double distilled or de-ionized water is use to prepare it. Main components of PSS are sodium (Na^+), chloride (Cl^-), potassium (K^+), magnesium (Mg^+), calcium (Ca^+) and glucose.

Most commonly used PSS:
• **Frog Ringer:** Rectus abdominus of frog
• **Tyrode:** Guinea pig ileum
• **De-Jalon:** Rat uterus
• **Krebs solution:** Rat fundus

Composition and Their Functions

• **Sodium:** Maintain the osmolarity, isotonicity, excitability and contractility.

TABLE 6.1: Composition of different types of PSS

Contents	Frog Ringer	Ringer locke	De Jalon	Tyrode	Krebs
NaCl	6	9.0	9	8.0	6.9
KCl	0.14	0.42	0.42	0.2	0.35
$CaCl_2$	0.12	0.24	0.06	0.2	0.28
$MgCl_2$	—	—	—	0.10	—
$MgSO_4$	—	—	—	—	1.28
$NaHCO_3$	0.2	0.5	0.5	1.0	2.1
NaH_2PO_4	—	—	—	0.05	—
KH_2PO_4	—	—	—	—	0.16
Glucose	2	1.0	0.5	1 or 2	1 or 2

All values are in g/L.

- **Potassium:** Nerve conduction and muscle contraction.
- **Calcium chloride:** Excitation of muscle, nerve and muscle contraction and relaxation.
- **Magnesium chloride:** Neuromuscular transmission, reduction of spontaneous activity of tissue.
- **Sodium bicarbonate:** Provide alkaline pH
- **Sodium and potassium di-hydrogen phosphate:** Acts as a buffer
- **Glucose:** Essential for energy requirements
- **Aeration:** O_2–100%, or carbogen—95% plus 5% CO_2

Important Precautions to be Taken While Making PSS

1. Calcium chloride combines with the bicarbonate of PSS leading to precipitation/chelation of the bicarbonate. This makes the solution turbid leading to reduction in the visibility of tissue in internal organ bath. This may change the property of PSS. To prevent this it should be added at the end.
2. The pH of PSS should be at the range of 7.3–7.4.
3. **Tyrode:** Non-innervated muscle and Krebs—nerve muscle preparation.
4. $MgCl_2$ can be replaced by $MgSO_4$ as later is not hygroscopic in nature, sulphate ions are not harmful and requirement of chloride ions can be fulfilled by NaCI.
5. Allowable error while making PSS should not be more than 1%.

Flowchart 6.1

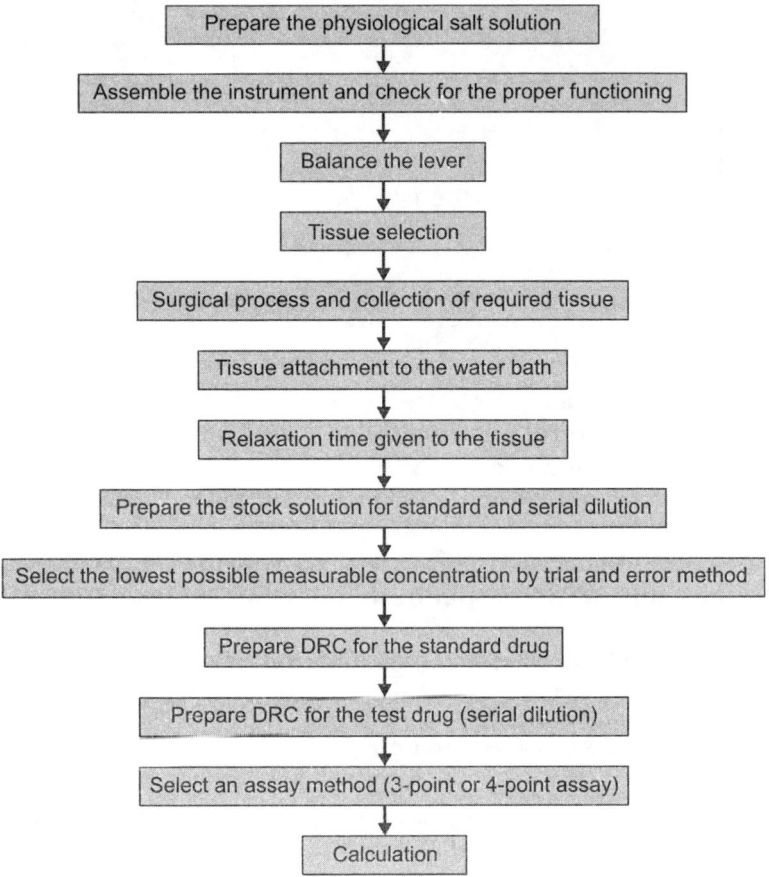

6. Calcium chloride and magnesium chloride should be added in stock solution because of their hygroscopic nature.

7. **PSS solution:** It is always prepared freshly to prevent the contamination by microbes. It can be stored for 24 hours in the refrigerator. Calcium and glucose should be added at the time of experiment. It is better to be prepared in the volume of 5 litre.

8. Aeration can be provided by oxygen, O_2 (100%) or 95% O_2 + 5% CO_2 which is called carbogen.

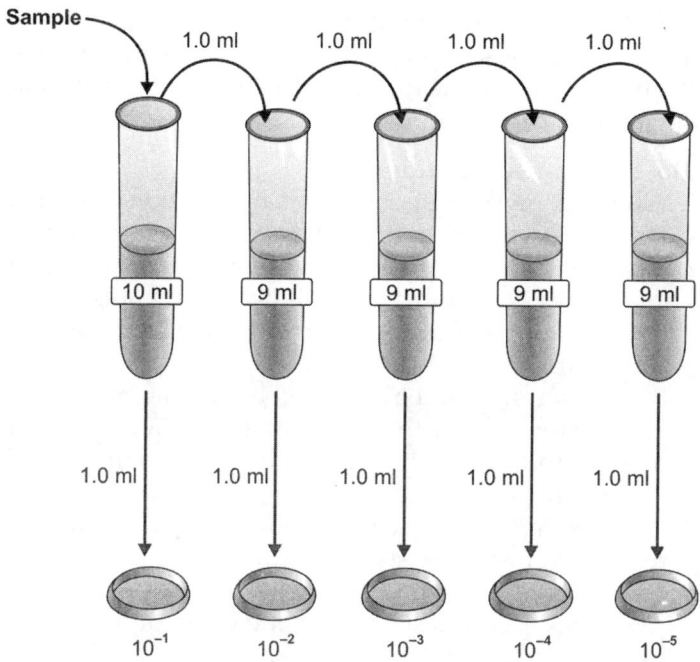

Fig. 6.3: Procedure for preparation of standard drug solution (serial dilution)

9. It is important to maintain the temperature of bath solution at a specified level to get a consistent effect. When temperature is reduced below 37°C intestinal tone may increase, this can vary the contraction and relaxation time It also reduces the height of contraction.

Important Features of Individual PSS

1. **Frog Ringer, Ringer locke and De Jalon:** No phosphate and magnesium ion
2. **McEwen:** Additional sucrose
3. **Aeration as carbogen:** Krebs, De Jalon, McEwen
4. **Use:** Krebs—for any tissue
   * Tyrode—smooth muscle (mammalian)
   * Heart muscle—Ringer Locke
   * Amphibian—frog Ringer
5. **Frog Ringer:** 400 ml distilled water + 1 litre Ringer locke

Serial dilution: To 1 ml of stock solution, add 9 ml of distil water. This is done subsequently in a similar manner as shown in the figure to reach the dilution of 10–9. This is applicable for standard and test solution.

Dose Response Relationship

1. While taking the response the concentration is marked on X-axis and the corresponding response is plotted on Y-axis.
2. We use log dose response curve or the doses are marked on logarithmic scale. It has the following advantages.
   a. Wide range of drug dose can be easily displayed on a graph.
   b. Graph can be accommodated on small graph paper.
   c. Easy to compare the potency and efficacy of agonist
   d. Easy to find out the competitive and noncompetitive antagonist.
3. It is a common practice of making ascending order dose response curve (i.e. start from low dose and increase it gradually). Descending order DRC can cause loss of tissue sensitivity. Intermittent higher and lower doses can also be used.
4. DRC of standard and test should be parallel

Various Methods Used for Bioassay Analysis

- Direct end point assay
- **Graded assay:** Matching, bracketing, interpolation, multiple point assay.

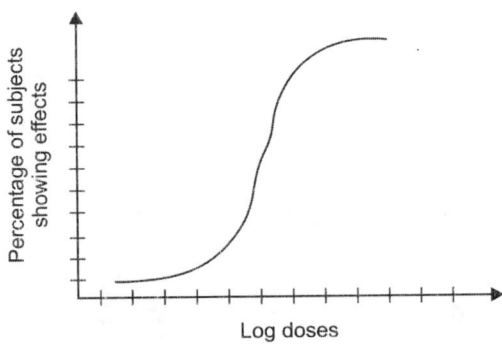

Log doses

Fig. 6.4: Quantal dose response curve

1. Direct Endpoint/quantal

Elicits an 'all or none' response in different animals, e.g. digitalis induced cardiac arrest in guinea pigs, hypoglycaemic convulsions in mice, D-Tc induced head drop in rabbits.

Procedure: In this method threshold dose, i.e. dose required for obtaining the predetermined response is calculated for standard and test drug.

By using the following formula strength/concentration of test drug is calculated.

- *Threshold dose standard (TDS):* Dose of standard required to achieve response.
- *Threshold dose test (TDT):* Dose of standard required to achieve response.
- *CSD:* Concentration of standard drug

$$\text{Concentration of test} = \frac{\text{TDS}}{\text{TDT}} \times \text{CSD}$$

Advantage: This method is rapid end-point detection.

Disadvantage: Only toxicity study or high dose study is possible and dose ranging study cannot be done.

Graded Response Assay

This can be done by various methods like:
- Matching
- Bracketing
- Interpolation
- *Multiple point assay:* Three point, four point and six point. This method is called graded response assay because the responses to varying doses of standard and test drug is measured on same tissue in a graded form, e.g. histamine on guinea pig ileum, acetylcholine on frog rectus.

Concentration of test can be obtained by any of the following methods:

Matching

In this method the response of test/unknown solution is matched with the response of the standard solution by trial and error method. From this finally the concentration of the test/ unknown solution is obtained.

Advantages
- This method is used when sample is small in amount.
- There is no need of making DRC of unknown solution, as only one dose which matches in response with standard is required.
- Simple and less time consuming

Disadvantages
- Tissue has to be very sensitive, hence tissue selection is an important aspect.
- Parallelism of dose response relationship is not ruled out (no DRC of unknown), hence experimental errors are not ruled out.

Formula

Concentration of T = Dose of S/Dose of T × conc. of S
where S: Standard and T: Test/unknown
Dose of standard: Log (volume of solution × dilution)

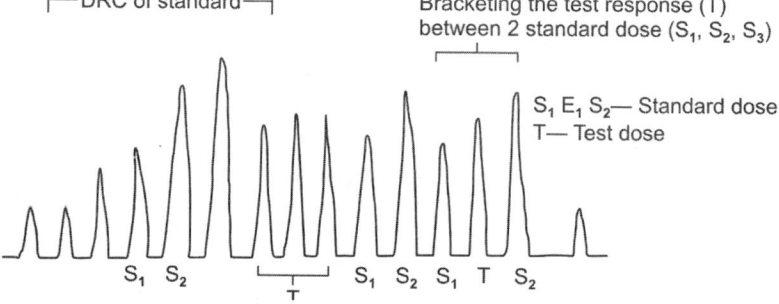

Fig. 6.5: Bracketing assay

Bracketing

In this method the observed response of test drug (T) is bracketed between the one smaller (S_1) and one larger (S_2) response of standard drug, hence it is called bracketing. Initially single or a few responses of test drug from any concentration is taken. Then the concentration of test is calculated directly from concentration of standard drug or by interpolation through dose response curve.

Advantages: Simple and can be used when test sample volume it too small.

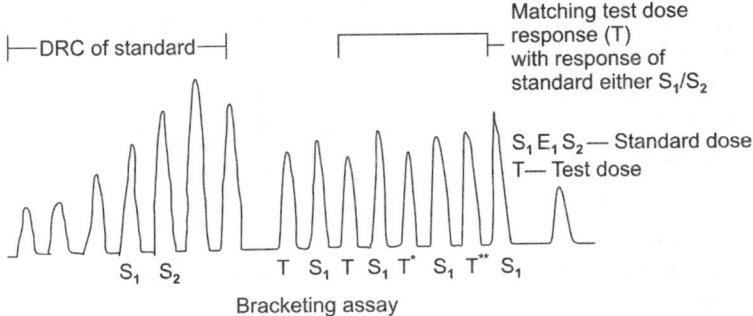

Bracketing assay

Fig. 6.6

Interpolation

This method depends on the principle of dose response curve. DRC of the standard drug is obtained

↓

Two doses of standard S_1 and S_2 is selected which fall in linear portion of DRC

↓

Then by trial and error 2 or 3 responses of test drug is found out which fall in linear portion of DRC

↓

Interpolate the response of test on the DRC of standard (Interpolate by drawing the perpendicular)

↓

Find out the concentration by antilog as shown in figure

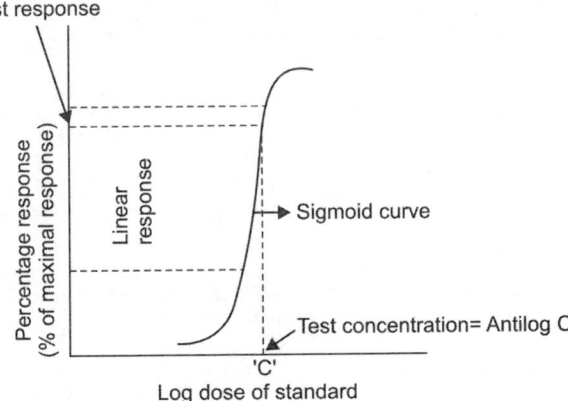

Fig. 6.7

Drawback: Poor precision and reliability and also unable to calculate error.

The above mentioned methods are not reliable and lack in sensitivity, accuracy because they do not take into account.

1. Changing tissue sensitivity with respect to time
2. Timing of the doses
3. Experimental errors

Hence graded response assays are preferred.

Multiple point assays

In this method 1 or more dose responses of test compound are selected

(Test doses must be in the linear portion of the DRC of standard compound, i.e. between 25 and 75%)

↓

These responses are compared with 2 or more responses of standards.

Advantages of multiple point assay: Repeated response recording in graded response assays minimize the tissue sensitivity error and improve the methodological errors.

Three-point assay

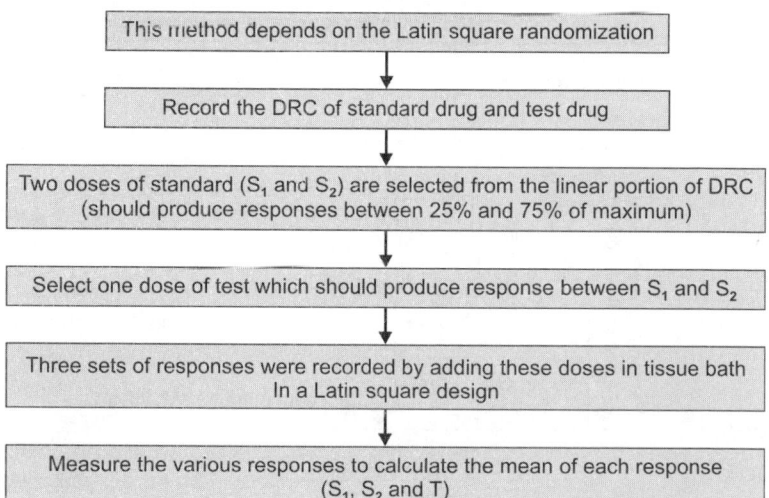

Latin square randomization

S$_1$	S$_2$	T
S$_2$	T	S$_1$
T	S$_1$	S$_2$

Calculation for 3-point assay:

$$\text{Relative potency } (M) = \frac{T - S_1}{S_2 - S_1} \times \log\left(\frac{S_2}{S_1}\right)$$

$$\text{Concentration of unknown compound} = \left(\frac{S_2}{S_1}\right) \times \text{antilog } M$$

= x times more concentrated than standard compound
where,

S$_1$ and S$_2$ = Length of standard dose response selected between 25 and 75%

T = Length of test dose response selected in between of two standard responses

s$_1$ and s$_2$ = Standard drug dose which came in contact with tissue and given the response S$_1$ and S$_2$ respectively

t = Test drug dose which came in contact with tissue and given the response T

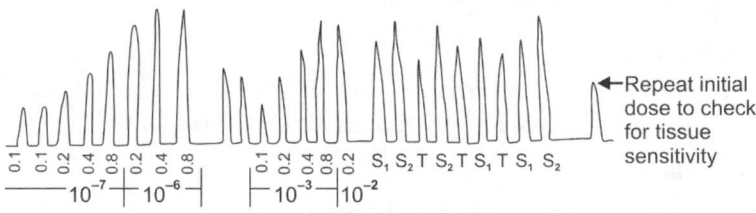

Fig. 6.8: Three-point assay

Four-point assay

Procedure is exactly same as that of three-point assay. The Latin square randomization table will be as follows.

S_1	S_2	T_1	T_2
S_2	T_1	T_2	S_1
T_1	T_2	S_1	S_2
T_2	S_1	S_2	T_1

$$M = S_2 - T_2 + S_1 - T_1 / S_2 - S_1 + T_2 - T_1 \times \text{Log of } s_2/s_1$$

S_1 and S_2 = Length of the standard dose response selected

T_1 and T_2 = Length of the test dose response selected

s_1 and s_2 = Doses which produce mean response of S_1 and S_2 respectively

t_1 and t_2 = Doses which produce mean response of T_1 and T_2 respectively

Concentration of unknown = $(s_1/t_1) \times$ antilog of M

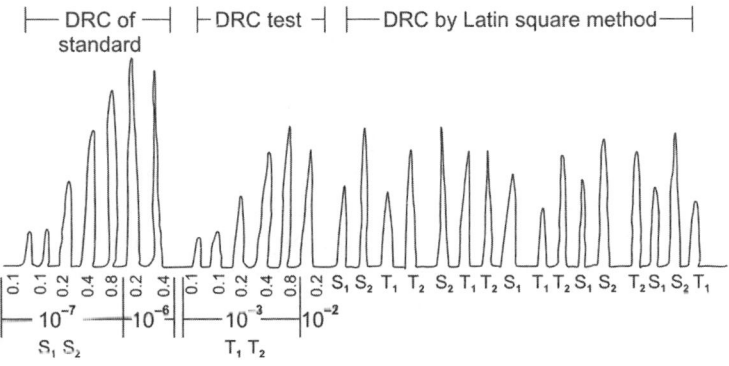

Fig. 6.9: Four-point assay

LEVERS IN EXPERIMENTAL PHARMACOLOGY

Writing Lever

It is the mechanical instrument used for recording and measuring the tissue length on a kymograph paper.

Materials

Aluminium, stainless steel, light balsum wood

Characteristics

- Light weight
- Fine
- Rigid to avoid bending while recording response.

Parts of a Lever

1. **Effort arm (E):** Force is applied here (tissue attachment).
2. **Load arm (L):** Where response is recorded.
3. **Fulcrum:** Point from which distance is calculated for load arm and effort arm
4. **Stylus:** Writing point on the lever

Depending on relative position of effort arm, load arm, fulcrum (as shown in Fig. 6.10a to c)

1. Fulcrum is in centre of load arm and effort arm, e.g. see-saw, scissors, bioassay lever.

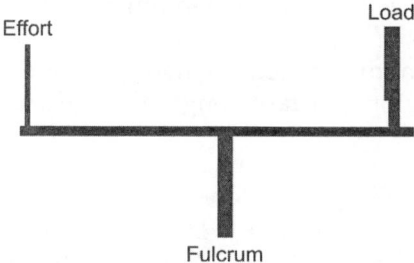

Fig. 6.10a: Type of 1 lever

2. Fulcrum at one end and effort at another. Load is at the centre, e.g. bottle opener.

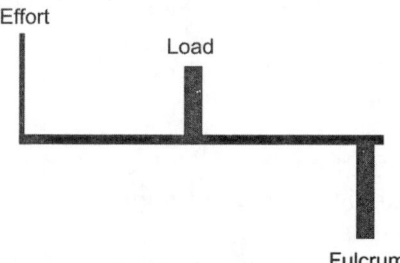

Fig. 6.10b: Type of 2 lever

3. Fulcrum and load arm are at either end or effort in the middle, e.g. forceps.

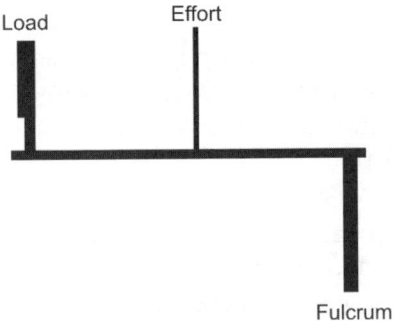

Fig. 6.10c: Type of 3 lever

Levers are also classified depending on the change in tissue length and tension.

Isometric: Length constant, change in tension

Isotonic: Tension constant, length change (guinea pig ileum bioassay)

Magnification (Mx)

It is defined as ratio of distance between fulcrum and writing point to the distance between fulcrum and tissue attachment.

Magnification (Mx) = A/B

A = distance between fulcrum and writing point

B = distance between fulcrum and tissue attachment

- It varies from tissue to tissue
- Depends on the inherent contractility of the tissue and nature of contraction (slow or rapidly contracting tissue), e.g.
  - Rapid contracting—
    - Ileum: 5–10
    - Uterus: 5
  - Slow contracting
    - Rat phrenic nerve diaphragm: 10–20
    - Frog rectus: 10

Depending on the position of stylus and kymograph paper, that is tangential or perpendicular, there are following types of lever.

Examples of lever:

- Simple lever: Attachment is tangential to drum

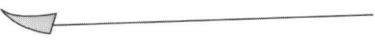

Simple lever

- Frontal writing lever: It has two arms which are perpendicular to the drum. Used for magnification.

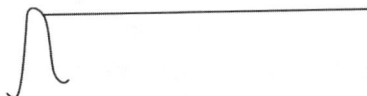

Frontal writing lever

- Starling heart lever: It has a metal frame, stylus is detachable.

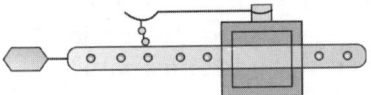

Starling heart lever

- Universal (Brodie's) lever
- Gimbal lever

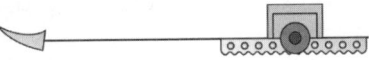

Gimbal lever

- Sprung lever

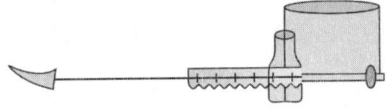

Sprung lever

- Auxotonic lever (Paton)

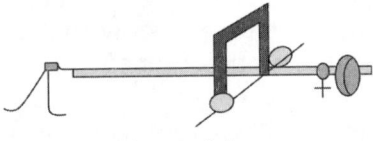

Auxotonic lever

- Torsion lever

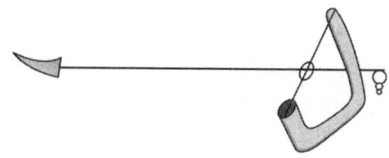

Torsion lever

Other Important Questions from Bioassay

Q1. What is the purpose of coil in organ bath?

Ans. To maintain PSS (physiological salt solution) for some time so that it is heated before reaching the inner bath.

Q2. What are the contents of outer and inner bath?

Ans. Outer bath—normal tap water
Inner bath—pss (tyrodes solution)

Q3. Why there is water in outer bath?

Ans. To maintain ideal temperature in inner tissue bath.

Q4. If it was a frog rectus, what temperature will be maintained?

Ans. Room temperature because it is amphibian and is poikilothermic.

Q5. What is the function of aerator-cum-tissue holder?
- To hold the tissue
- Aeration of the tissue
- Mixing of the drug

Q6. What solvent is used to make tyrodes solution?

Ans. Double distilled water

Q7. What are the different types of muscle contraction?

Ans. Isometric—length is same, tone changes, e.g. skeletal muscle twitch
Isotonic—tone same, length changes, e.g. guinea pig ileum contraction

Q8. What is the tone/tension here and why is it required?

Ans. 0.5–1 gm. It is needed to stabilize the tissue and increase the readiness of the tissue to contract.

Q9. Give examples of fast and slow contracting tissues.

Ans. Fast contacting tissue—guinea pig/rat ileum, colon, rat uterus.
Slow contacting tissue—frog rectus abdominis muscle, guinea pig tracheal chain.

Q10. Why experiment started after a lag period?

Ans. To give time for the tissue to acclimatize.

Q11. What is the rate of aeration?

Ans. 10–12 bubbles per minute.

Q12. Why is guinea pig fasted overnight with only water and libitum?

Ans. To decrease the intestinal faecal matter.

Q13. How is guinea pig sacrificed?

Ans. Stunning/sudden neck jerking and cut the neck vessels to cause early death.

Q14. How do you identify ileum?

Ans. By identifying ileocaecal junction. Leaving around 10 cm of terminal ileum tissue pieces are taken of lengh 2–3 cm.

Q15. How is the tissue washed and cut?

Ans. Washing should be done from proximal to distal direction as that is the normal peristaltic movement in intestines and receptors are not damaged. To mark the proximal part keep it outside petridish while washing by tyrodes filled pipette inclined at an angle. (Do not blow—tissue gets stretched and receptors damaged.) Warm tyrode from inner tissue bath. Tissue is washed first before cutting into 2–3 cm pieces to avoid tissue damage. The mesentry attatched to ileum is cut by corneal/mosquito scissor.

Q16. What is dose cycle?

Ans. It is 3 minutes cycle, start drum and let it rotate for 30 seconds, add drug and let the rotation continue. Stop the drug and wait for 2 minutes. Give a wash to the inner tissue bath in the mean time.

BIBLIOGRAPHY

1. HL Sharma and KK Sharma, Principles of Pharmacology, 2nd edition 2011, Paras publication, Bioassay of drugs, 921–926.
2. Medhi B, Prakash A. Practical manual of clinical and experimental Pharmacology, Chapter No. 02 Bioassay, New Dehli, Jaypee Brothers Medical Publication, Second edition 2017.
3. Sunil J Panujanty, Principle involved in bioassay by different methods: A mini review, Research and reviews: research journal of biology, Vol:3, Issue:2, 2015, 1–18.

Short Experiments

Objective

To study the effect of chlorpromazine on spontaneous motor activity in mice by using actophotometer.

Principle

Drugs acting on CNS also influence the locomotor activity in man and animals.

Most of the CNS acting drugs influence the locomotor activities in man and animals. The CNS depressant drugs such as barbiturates and alcohol reduce the motor activity while the stimulants such as caffeine and amphetamines increase the activity. In other words, the locomotor activity can be an index of wakefulness (alertness) of mental activity. The locomotor activity can be easily measured using an actophotometer which operates on photoelectric cells which are connected in circuit with a counter. When the beam of light falling on the photo cell is cut off by the animal, a count is recorded on the digital display. An actophotometer could have either circular or square area in which the animal moves. Both rats and mice may be used for testing in this equipment.

Experimental Animal: Rat/mice

Equipment: Actophotometer

Drugs: Test (drug under evaluation) and control (NS 0.9%)

Procedure

Step 1: Select male mice with approximately 20–25 g.

Step 2: Divide them in two groups, test and control.

Step 3: Turn on the equipment and place individually each mouse in the activity cage for 10 minutes. Note the basal activity score of all the animals.

Step 4: Administer NS 0.2 ml ip in control.

Step 5: Inject chlorpromazine (Dose: 3 mg/kg, ip) in test group

Step 6: After 30 minutes re-test the activity in both the groups.

Step 7: Calculate percent decrease in motor activity.

Commonly Used Drugs

CNS Depressants

- Chlorpromazine hydrochloride   (3 mg/kg, ip in case of both rat and mice)
- Fluoxetine   (10 mg/kg, ip in case of rat)
- Imipramine   (10–20 mg/kg, ip in case both mice and rat)
- Phenobarbitone sodium   (10 mg/kg, ip in case of both rat and mice)
- Alcohol   (0.5–2 g, ip, po in case of both mouse and rat)

CNS Stimulants

Caffeine   (8–10 mg/kg, ip in case of mice and 30 mg/kg, ip in case of rat)

Amphetamine   (1.5 mg/kg, ip in case of mice and 3–5 mg/kg, sc, ip in case of rat)

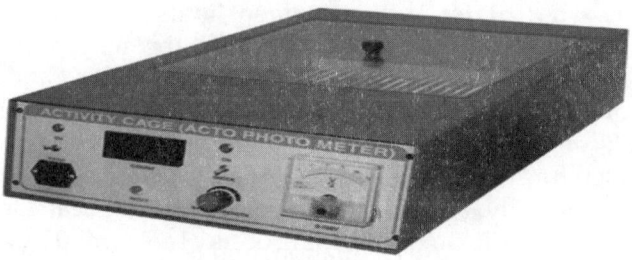

Fig. 7.1: Actophotometer

Results

S. No	Body weight	Treatment	Dose (mg/kg)	Locomotor activity in 10 min before drug, after drug
1. Control group				
2. Test group				

Inference

• Reduction in the motor activity indicates CNS depressant property of the drug.
• Increase in the motor activity indicates CNS stimulant property of the drug.

DEMONSTRATE ANALGESIC ACTIVITY OF DRUG BY USING TAIL–FLICK/HOT PLATE ANALGESIOMETER

Objective

To study the analgesic effect of morphine by using tail-flick/hot plate analgesiometer.

Principle

Analgesic activity of the test compound is evaluated by observing the change in reaction time in response to pain. Increase in reaction time indicates analgesic activity of the drug. In this method heat is used as a stimulus to induce the pain.

Tail-flick/hot plate analgesiometer is used for evaluation of narcotic analgesics (acts through central mechanism)

Eddy's hot plate: This instrument is used for evaluation of non-narcotic analgesics which acts through peripheral mechanism.

It consists of the hot plate, which is commercially available, consists of a electrically heated surface. The temperature is controlled for 55° to 56°C. This can be a copper plate or a heated glass surface. The animals are placed on the hot plate and the time until either licking or jumping occurs is recorded by a stop-watch.

Requirements

Animal   : Albino rats (150–200 g) of either sex
Drugs   : Pethidine 30 mg/kg/SC
              Normal saline, 0.9% w/v NaCl solution.
Equipment : Tail-flick/**hot plate** analgesiometer

Procedure

Step 1: Weigh the animals, divide them into 2 groups and mark them control and test group.

Step 2: Measure the basal reaction time to radiant heat by placing the tip of the tail (last 1–2 cm) on the radiant heat source. End point is tail flicking time. Normally a rat withdraws its tail within 3–5 seconds. Cut off time for mice is 15–20 seconds, in case of rat it is 20–30 seconds. This is to prevent the damage to the tail.

Step 3: Inject normal saline to the control group and pethidine to the test group in the specified dose and note the reaction time after 30, 60, 90 and 120 minutes of drug administration.

Step 4: Calculate percentage increase in reaction time (index of analgesia) at each time interval.

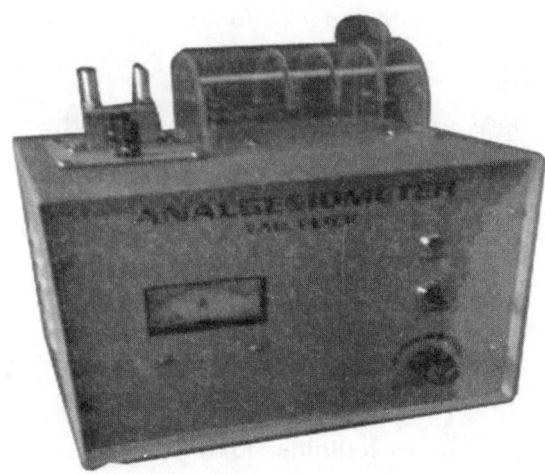

Fig. 7.2: Tail-flick analgesiometer

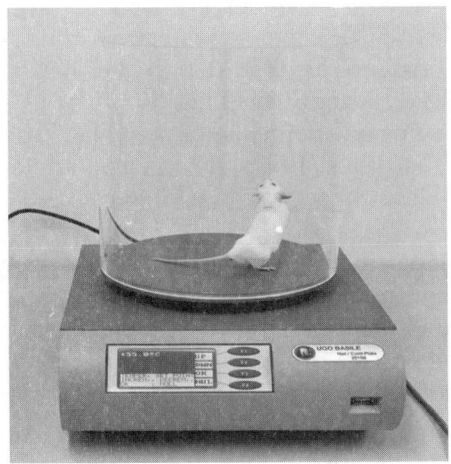

Fig. 7.3: Eddy's hot plate

Inference

Increase reaction time in the test group indicates analgesic activity of the compound which acts through central mechanism.

EFFECT OF DRUGS ON RABBIT EYE

Objective: To study the effects of various drugs on rabbit eye.

Background

Miotics: These are the drugs which constrict the pupil. This is because of contraction of circular muscle fibres of iris (constrictor pupillae).

Mydriatics: These are the drugs which dilate the pupil. This is because of two reasons:
  a. Contraction of radial muscle fibres of iris (dilator pupillae)—active mydriasis
  b. Paralysis of circular muscle fibers—passive mydriasis

Receptors and Pathways Involved

Circular muscle fibres contains M3 muscarinic receptors. Their activation results in miosis. Radial muscle fibres contain α_1 adrenergic which have role in mydriasis.

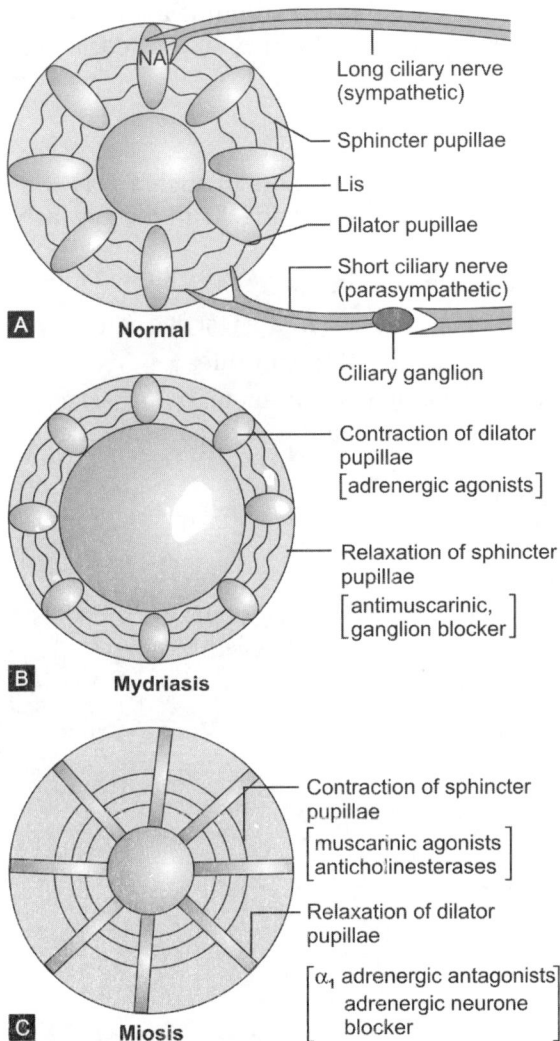

Fig. 7.4: Effect of different drugs on pupil size

Requirements

Experimental Animal: Rabbits.

Equipment: Dropper, rabbit restrainer, pupillometer, torch

Drugs: Adrenaline 0.1%, physostigmine 2%, atropine, homatropine 0.5%, ephedrine 5%, pilocarpine 0.5%, cocaine 1%, guanethidine 5%

Procedure

Step 1: Put the rabbits in holders in such a way that the head will be protruding outside. Trim the eye lashes of both the eyes.

Step 2: Mark test and control eye.

Step 3: Instill drug solution in the test eye carefully.

Step 4: Study the effect after 5 minutes.

Step 5: Note the following parameters: Pupil size, response to light (light reflex) and touch (corneal reflex).

Visual Pathway

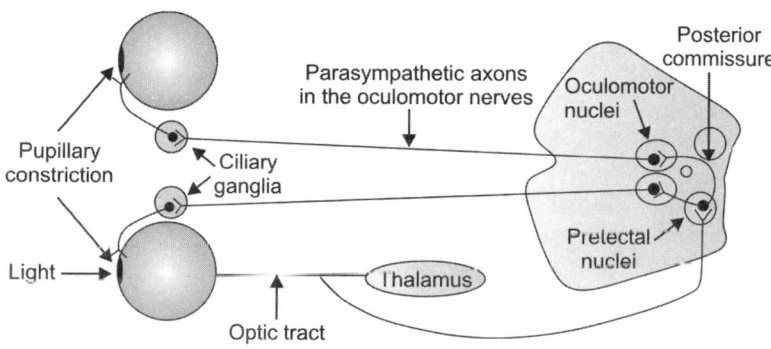

Fig. 7.5: Visual pathway

Results

Sl No.	Drugs	Papillary size	Light reflex	Corneal reflex
1.	Saline	Normal	Present	Present
2.	Physostigmine/pilocarpine	Constriction	Present	Present
3.	Cocaine	Dilation	Present	Absent
4.	Phenylephrine	Dilation	Present	Present
5.	Atropine	Dilation	Absent	Present

Discussion

1. Pilocarpine is a directly acting parasympathomimetic agent.
2. Physostigmine is an anti-cholinesterase agent (indirectly acting parasympathomimetic agent). Both the drugs can be absorbed locally and produce miosis.
3. Morphine is not absorbed locally and hence effect is not observed. However, if given intravenously, it stimulates Edinger-Westphal nucleus in the brain and results in pinpoint pupils.
4. Ephedrine is an indirectly acting sympathomimetic agent. It produces mydriasis. The light reflex and corneal reflex are not affected by ephedrine.
5. Cocaine is a local anaesthetics agent, hence corneal reflexes are lost if cocaine is instilled. The mydriatic action of cocaine is due to its noradrenaline uptake blocking activity. Since neither uptake of noradrenaline is blocked, more noradrenaline is available at the site to produce mydriasis.
6. Atropine blocks the muscarine receptors, hence the sympathetic system predominates, resulting in mydriasis. Since parasympathetic responses are abolished—cyclopegia (loss of accommodation).

ROTAROD APPARATUS

Principle

The rotarod, also known as the rotarod test, is used as a basic assessment tool for coordination and balance in rodents and provides one measure of locomotor ability. Animals with deficits affecting balance or coordination fall from the apparatus more quickly than animals with normal motor function.

Apparatus

The rotarod apparatus consists of a rotating cylinder, typically 3–3.5 cm in diameter for mice and 7–7.5 cm in diameter for rats. The cylinder is usually made of a solid material such as rubber. The rotation of the rod nowadays is motor-driven. Many rotarod devices are designed to accommodate simultaneous testing of multiple subjects. The cylinder is mounted above a platform, typically at a height of 15 cm for mice and 30 cm for rats. Devices may also be equipped with timers that allow for automatic recording of time from start of the test to when the animal contacts the platform.

Benzodiazepines (diazepam) are the most popular sedative and hypnotic agents. These drugs have taming/calming effect together with muscle relaxant action. This effect can be easily studied in animals by using rotarod/inclined plane.

Parameter for Observation

The difference in the fall off time from the rotating rod between the control group and test group.

Requirements

- **Experimental animals:** Mice
- **Drugs:** Normal saline (NS), drug under evaluation (test), standard drug like diazepam
- **Equipment:** Rotarod
- **Procedure:**
  1. Weigh the animals and number them
  2. Divide them in control (A) and test (B) group (minimum 4 in each group)
  3. Turn on rotarod and select the appropriate speed (12 rev./min.)
  4. Place the animal one by one on the rotating rod. Note down the 'fall of time' for each animal. (Generally normal mouse falls off within 3–5 minutes)
  5. Administered the test drug and control (NS) by subcutaneous/oral route.
  6. Post-treatment again measures the score (no. of fall and duration of performance) in all animals.

Results

Increase number of falls and reduce period of performance suggest that the drug has either CNS depressant/skeletal muscle property.

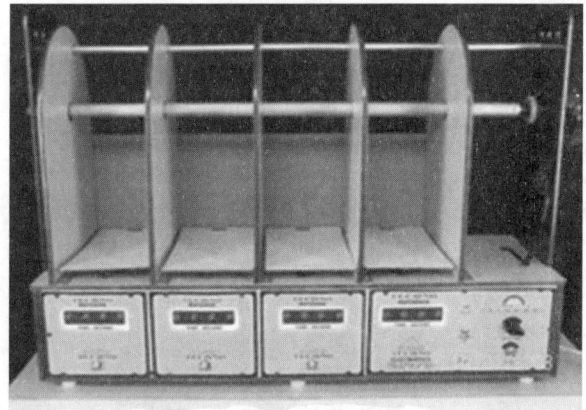

Fig. 7.6: Rotarod apparatus

ELECTROCONVULSIOMETER

Principle

To study the antiepileptic effect of the drugs by using electro-convulsiometer

Materials and Methods

- **Experimental Animal:** Rat/Mouse (150–250 gm)
- **Drugs:**
  - Phenytoin   : 20–30 mg/kg, ip/po
  - Phenobarbitone sodium : 15 mg/kg, ip
  - Diazepam   : 3–4 mg/kg, ip
- **Instrument:** Electroconvulsiometer
  Electric shock
  - *Rat:* 150 mA, 50 Hz for 0.2 sec
  - *Mouse:* 12 mA, 50 Hz for 0.2 sec

Procedure

- **Step 1**
  - Weight the animals and mark properly
  - Divide animals into 3 groups
  - They are given stimulus with ear electrode.
  - Phases of convulsions are recorded in each mouse
  - The drugs are injected.

- **Step 2**
  - *Group 1:* Isotonic saline
  - *Group 2:* Phenytoin sodium, 30 mg/kg, ip
  - *Group 3:* Phenobarbitone sodium, 15 mg/kg, ip

  After 1 hour animals are given electroconvulsions
  - Observations are noted
  - Record whether THLE (tonic high limb extension) present/absent

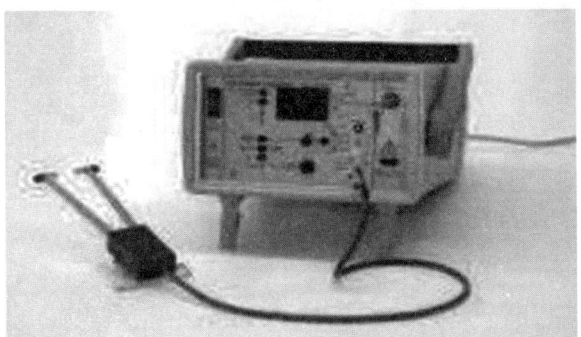

Fig. 7.7: Electroconvulsiometer

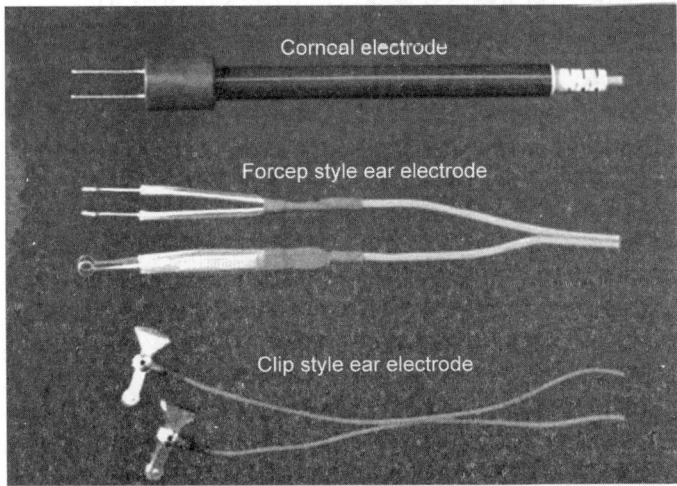

Fig. 7.8: Corneal and ear electrode

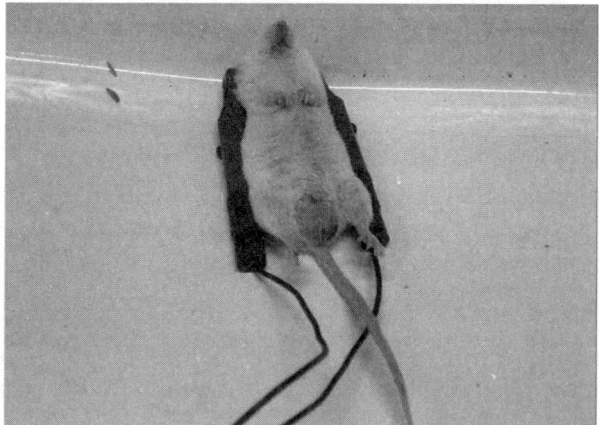

Fig. 7.9: Tonic hind limb extension

- **Step 3**
  - Observe the animal after MES
  - Calculate percentage protection
  - Percentage protection = No. of animals with THLE absent / total no. of animals ×100

TO DEMONSTRATE THE STRAUB TAIL PHENOMENON INDUCED BY MORPHINE

Background

Straub tail means erected tail. The phenomenon was used to check doping, i.e. opioid level in the horses which took part in the race.

Principle

Straub tail reaction is due to mechanical contraction of the dorsal sacrococcygeus muscle and electrical stimulation of spinal cord. Dorsal sacrococcygeus muscle is present on either side of the tail and originating at the base of spinal cord. Various studies suggest that straub tail results because of direct action on the opioids μ-receptor, most important μ_2–receptor. There are some studies which suggest that it also results through 5-HT receptors, α_2-(alpha-2) receptors, dopamine receptors and glucocorticoid receptors as well.

Procedure

A subcutaneous injection of morphine hydrochloride (10–40 mg/kg, ip/sc) is given into the mouse flank.

Response

This produces 'S'-shape erection of the tail within 2 to 5 minutes after the injection, depending on the dose. Finally, the tail curves back along the body of the animal, the tip touching the centre of the head.

Straub tail phenomenon can also be seen with injection of the centrally acting analgesics such as opioids. But, there are no such studies which have supporting data for the peripheral analgesic induced straub tail.

Materials and Methods

Materials

Animal/species	:	Mice/albino Swiss
Sex/body weight	:	Male/20–30 g
Syringe/needle	:	1 ml/preferably 24G onwards
Drug	:	Morphine (10–40 mg/kg, sc or ip)

Precautions Before Experimentation

- Animals should be marked properly, to avoid mixing in two groups
- Handle the animal with care (minimize the stress and pain to animal)
- Observe the animal in a plexiglass chamber
- Laboratory should be noise free (noise may delay the response).

Methods

- **Step 1**
  - Weigh the animals and mark into test and control groups.
  - Divide animals into two groups (n = 6 in each group).
- **Step 2**
  - *Group 1:* Control group (n = 6); mice are given the saline at the equivalent dose of drug
  - *Group 2:* Treatment group (n = 6); mice are given morphine at the dose of 40 mg/kg, sc

- **Step 3**
  - Observe the animals for 45 min in plexiglass chamber
  - Observe the animals behaviour carefully, for (1) onset of straub tail reaction/phenomenon, (2) duration of straub tail reaction and (3) any additional behaviour changes.

Results

Numerical score for straub tail reaction/phenomenon

The tail rise at an angle >30° is considered to be the positive straub tail reaction. There is no clinical condition resembling this condition, hence have only experimental implication.

0 = 0	0.5 = 1–30	1 = 31–45	1.5 = 46–60	2.0 = 61–90	2.5 = more than 90

COOK'S POLE CLIMBING TEST/CONDITIONED AVOIDANCE RESPONSE (CAR)

Principle

Cook's Pole Climbing Apparatus use to study cognitive function, mainly a response to conditioned stimuli during learning and its retention.

The apparatus has an experimental chamber ($25 \times 25 \times 25$ cm) with the floor grid in a soundproof enclosure. Scrambled shock (6 mA) is delivered to the grid floor of the chamber composed of stainless steel rods. A pole, 2.5 cm in diameter, hangs inside the chamber through a hole in the upper centre of the chamber.

Procedure

Step 1: The is placed in the chamber and allowed to explore the chamber for 45 seconds.

Step 2: Conditioned stimulus—buzzer signal turned on unconditioned stimulus—electric shock delivered through grid floor for 45 Seconds

Step 3: Animal learned to associate the buzzer with the impending foot shock and is now capable of avoiding the foot shock by climbing the pole after buzzer signal.

Step 4: Avoidance response defined as climbing reaction time 10 sec.

Step 5: Training

Every rat is subjected to maximum 05 trials on 1st day, and 24 hours later, rat is subjected to relearning trials (2nd day 3 trials and on 3rd day one trial) and transfer latency is noted to check the retention of conditioned avoidance response (CAR) and escape response.

Animals are screened by using this model and those which demonstrate at least one escape response either on day one or two are included in the study.

This apparatus is used to differentiate between minor and major tranquilizers.

Minor Tranquilizer

• Most commonly used drug in psychopharmacology, e.g. benzodiazepines.
• They have CNS depressant and skeletal muscle relaxant property.

Major Tranquilizer

• Less commonly used, e.g. antipsychotics.
• Has only CNS depressant, no SMR action.

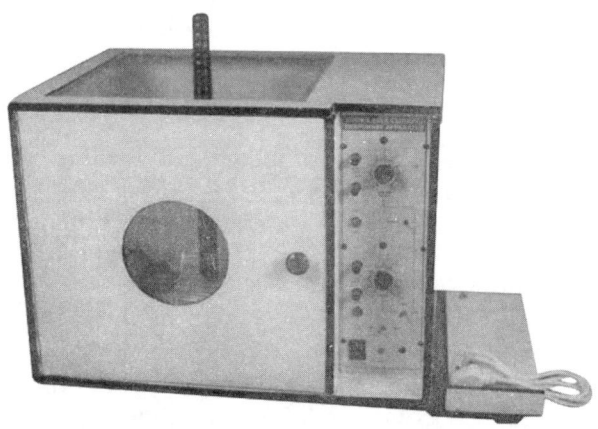

Fig. 7.10: Cook's pole climbing apparatus

Requirements

- **Experimental animals:** Trained rats.
- **Drugs:** Normal saline and test drug.
- **Equipment:** Cook's pole climbing apparatus.

Conditioned response: Animal will respond to both shock and buzzer.

Unconditioned response: Response to buzzer will be lost.

Results

Drugs	Avoidance response	
	Unconditioned	Conditioned
Normal saline	Present	Present
Minor tranquilizer	Absent	Absent
Major tranquilizer	Present	Absent

BIBLIOGRAPHY

1. Parle M, Yadav M, Labortory models for screening analgesics, International Journal of research Pharmacy, 2013, Vol. 4, Issue 1, Page 15–9.
2. Vogel HG et al, Drug discovery and evaluation: Methods in clinical Pharmacology, Germany, Springer Publication House.
3. YK Gupta et al. Methods and considerations for experimental evaluation of antiepileptic drugs. Indian J Physiol Pharmacol 1999; 43(1): 25–43

Therapeutic Drug Monitoring

Therapeutic drug monitoring (TDM) is the process of modifying a patient's drug therapy based on measurements of drug concentration achieved in biological fluids like blood, plasma, urine, etc. Measurement of plasma drug concentration can give an estimate of the pharmacokinetic variables in that patient and the magnitude of difference from an 'average patient', so that appropriate adjustments in the dosage regimen can be made.

Formula for calculating revised dosage regime:

Revised dose rate =

$$\text{Previous dose rate} \times \text{Target Cpss} / \text{Measured Cpss}$$

Requirements for TDM

- **Role of clinician:** To assess the need for TDM followed by that, if needed, alter the doses
- **Role of analytical technique:** Which can precisely measure drug concentration even in less sample
- **Role of skilled expert:** To operate the instrument and get proper output
- **Role of clinical pharmacologist:** Result is interpreted after co-ordinating with the patient history

Properties of a drug for which TDM is done:

- Drugs for which reliable clinical response is not measurable, e.g. antiepileptics and anticancer
- Drugs with narrow therapeutic index, e.g. lithium, digoxin, aminoglycosides

- Definite and predictable dose response relationship exists, e.g. theophylline (with increasing dose: Dyspepsia, headache, nervousness, tremors, vomiting, palpitations, tachypnea, flushing, hypotension, convulsions, shock, arrhythmias)
- Showing saturation and zero order kinetics—drug accumulates in the body when given in large doses. Theophylline, phenytoin.
- Reliable analytical techniques exists to measure the concentration of drugs, e.g. high performance liquid chromatography (HPLC), enzyme-linked immune sorbent assay (ELISA).
- Drugs which are used for extremely short duration
- If individual variations are large, e.g. antidepressants, lithium.

Purpose of Doing TDM

- Individualizing therapy:
  - ◆ Particularly required for narrow safety margin and drugs which follow zero order kinetics.
  - ◆ Patients with liver/kidney failure, e.g. vancomycin in renal failure patients.
- *Toxicity minimization:* This is required for highly toxic drugs like aminoglycosides, theophylline.
- Compliance monitoring, e.g. anticonvulsants, antipsychotic drugs.
- To monitor whether required effective plasma concentration is achieved or not when drug is given for prophylaxis, e.g. immunosuppresants for renal transplant patients and anti-epileptic for brain tumour patients.
- *To prevent under-treatment of patients:* Antibiotic resistance.
- *Confirming adverse drug-drug interaction:* When two nephrotoxic drugs vancomycin and aminoglycosides are given together.
- *Checking quality of the drug:* Spurious/substandard
- Guiding withdrawal of therapy, e.g. to stop digoxin if patient is stable even after low plasma levels of digoxin.
- Differentiating adverse drug reaction from disease progress.
- *Digoxin in CHF:* Toxicity will present with nausea vomiting and CHR deterioration also present with nausea and vomiting.

- Failure of response without any apparent reason, e.g. antimicrobials
- Poisoning cases
- To confirm drug abuse

Drugs Not Suitable for TDM

- Drugs that are used for treating diseases of which their clinical end points can easily be monitored, e.g. BP, HR, cardiac rhythm, blood sugar, blood cholesterol and triglycerides, urine volume, body temperature, pain, headache.
- Drugs whose serum concentrations do not correlate with therapeutic or toxic effects.
- Drugs with less complicated pharmacokinetics.
- Drugs having wide therapeutic index.
- Hit and run drugs: Omeprazole, MAO inhibitors.

Steps in TDM

1. Clinician assess the patients disease status and treatment to identify if TDM is required
2. Desired biological sample is collected.
3. A predesigned TDM request form is filled which contains detailed information of patient, disease, sample, drug and why TDM is required.
4. The sample is received by the TDM unit and is processed to run the test.
5. The sample is analyzed using appropriate analytical technique.
6. The results are interpreted by a clinical pharmacologist. The output data from tests and patient details are analyzed to give a recommendation to clinician.
7. Clinician orders a revised dosage regime for the patient.
8. The same steps may be repeated in case TDM is required again.

Important Considerations with TDM

- Where to find therapeutic range of drugs—package inserts and books like physician desk reference.
- Timing of sample collection:
  - *Trough samples for most drugs are taken:* 30 minutes before the next dose

- Usually a steady state concentration is measured
- *For highly toxic drugs:* Peak concentration taken, e.g. gentamycin.

- *Free drug concentration:* Important for drugs which are highly plasma protein bound, e.g. phenytoin.
- *Metabolites concentration:* The analytical technique may not differentiate the main drug and its metabolites.

Examples of drugs requiring TDM with their therapeutic range:

- Digoxin   : 0.8–2 µcg/L
- Theophylline : 10–20 mg/L
- Gentamicin   : 2–12 mg/L
- Lithium   : 0.8–1.2 mmol/L
- Phenytoin   : 10–20 mg/L
- Carbamazepine : 4–12 mg/L
- Ciclosporin   : 100–200 ng/ml
- Vancomycin : 10–20 mg/L

ANALYTICAL TECHNIQUES

Analytical technique is a method that is used to determine the concentration of a chemical compound or a chemical element in biological sample. It is very important to measure the concentration of drugs in the blood or plasma. They are used for therapeutic monitoring of drugs. The common analytical techniques are as follows:

High Performance Liquid Chromatography (HPLC)

It is also known as high pressure liquid chromatography. It is a type of column chromatography which is used to:
- Separate the components in a mixture
- Identify individual components
- Quantify individual components.

Principle

- Substances are separated depending on the relative distribution of mixture constituents in the two phases—mobile phase and a stationary phase.
- Substances distributed in mobile phase move through the column more rapidly than those in stationary phase.

Parts of the Equipment

- It contains two phases:
  - ◆ **Stationary phase:** Column made up of a solid adsorbent material, e.g. silica.
  - ◆ **Mobile phase:** Liquid solvent containing sample mixture, e.g. water, methanol, acetonitrile
- Pump: To force the liquid into the column
- Sample injector
- Detector
- Data processing unit

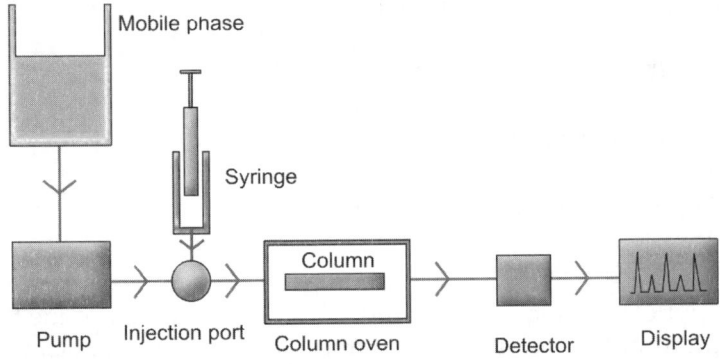

Fig. 8.1: HPLC

Variants of HPLC

- **Normal phase liquid chromatography:** Stationary phase or absorbent is used in the ionized form and mobile phase in unionized form
- **Reverse phase chromatography:** Stationary phase is used in unionized form and mobile phase in ionized form
- **Gel filtration chromatography:** Liquid/gas passes through a porous which separates the molecules depending upon its size
- **Ion exchange chromatography:** It allows the separation of ions and polar molecules based on their charge.

Uses

- Research
- TDM

- Detection of analytes in biological and non-biological samples
- Quality control tool in chemical, pharmaceutical, toxicological, cosmetics and food

Advantages
- Highly sensitive and specific
- Precise and accurate
- Standardized assays available for many drugs

Disadvantages
- Expensive
- Technical skill required
- Time consuming

RADIOIMMUNOASSAY (RIA)

An immunoassay is a technique that uses an antigen–antibody complex to generate a measurable response. RIA is an immunoassay which detects and measures antigen using a radioactive label. It was developed by Yalow and Berson in 1960 for insulin.

Principle
Competition between radiolabeled and unlabeled antigen (test sample) for the limited binding site on the specific antibody.

Requirements
- Radioactive labeled antigen.
- Specific antibody to the antigen to be measured.
- Various techniques to separate antigen–antibody complex, e.g. double antibody, charcoal, cellulose, chromatography.
- Instrument to measure radioactivity-gamma counter.
- Radioisotopes, e.g. I 125, I 131, H3

Procedure
- A measured quantity of labelled antigen is mixed with antibody which bind to each other.
- Unlabel antigen present in the sample is mixed with the solution.
- This leads to competition between the labelled and unlabelled antigen to occupy the antibody.

- This leads to release of certain amount of labelled antigens depending upon the concentration of unlabelled antigen in the sample.

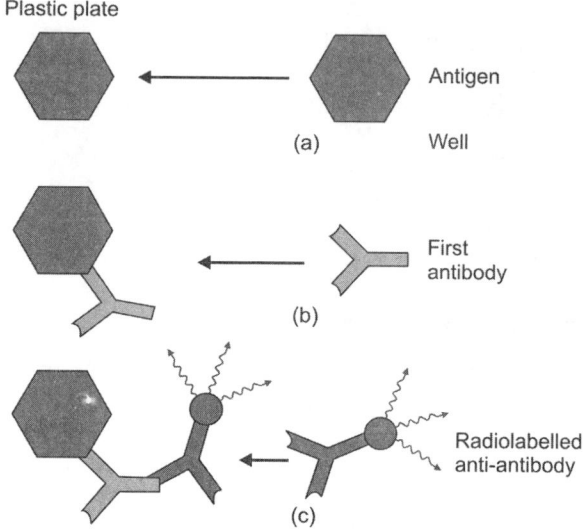

Fig. 8.2: Radioimmunoassay (RIA)

Uses

- Estimation of protein hormones and peptides
- TDM
- RAST (Radioallergosorbent test) to detect allergens

Advantages

- Sensitive and specific
- Less expensive
- Can measure very small molecules

Disadvantages

- Require specialized instrument
- Waste disposal hazard
- Special precaution and licensing
- Quality control and standards must be performed with each run.

ENZYME LINKED IMMUNOSORBENT ASSAY (ELISA)

It is an analytical technique that uses antibodies attached to an enzyme and then the colour change produced to detect a substance.

Procedure

- Sample with unknown amount of antigen is immobilized on a well
- A specific antibody linked to an enzyme is added which binds to the antigens
- A substrate is now added which reacts with the enzyme to produce a detectable signal (usually a colour change)
- The signal is measured by ELISA plate reader
  The enzymes and substrates commonly used are:
  - *Enzyme*: Horseradish peroxidase (HRP), alkaline phosphatase (AP).
  - Substrate-o-phenylenediamine (OPD) hydrochloride, p-nitrophenyl phosphate (PNPP) disodium salt.

Types of ELISA

- **Direct ELISA:** As explained above.
- **Indirect ELISA:** Enzyme is linked to secondary antibody.
- **Sandwich ELISA:** A separate antibody is used to stick the antigen in sample to the wall.

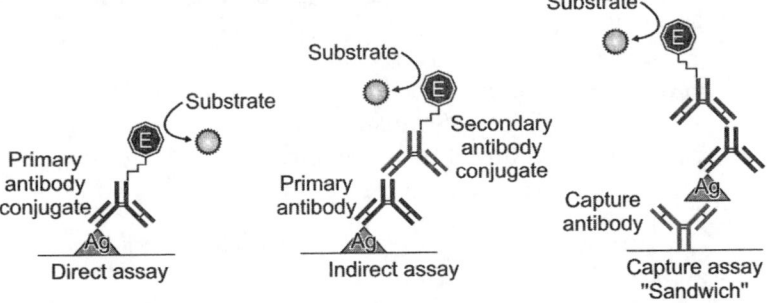

Fig. 8.3: Types of ELISA

Uses

- To diagnose diseases like HIV, hepatitis.
- Pregnancy hormones (HCG, LH).
- Drug allergens.

- TDM of various drugs.
- Screening of blood for HIV 1 and 2, hepatitis B and C.

Advantages

- High sensitivity and specificity.
- Large no. of samples can be processed at a time.
- No radiation hazard or waste disposal issue.
- Long shelf life of reagents.

Disadvantages

- False positive and false negative results are possible
- ELISA kits are costly
- Enzyme activity may be affected by plasma constituents

SPECTROPHOTOMETRY

Photometry

This principle is used to measure different substances having the capacity to absorb and reflect the light of different wavelengths.

Principle

Light is passed through a solution which has the capacity to absorb light of particular wavelength and the complementary light is reflected back.

A = amount of light absorbed called absorbance

It is calculated as

$A = -\log_{10} I/I_0 = kcl$

where I = intensity of incident light

       I_0 = intensity of transmitted light

       k = constant of the substance

       c = concentration

       l = length of light path

COLORIMETER

Procedure: This method measures the concentration of the coloured solution in the visible spectrum of light (300–750 nm) using a tungsten lamp. A colour filter is used to absorb and allow only the desired wavelength of light to pass through it. The intensity of emerging light is measured by photoelectric device attached to a galvanometer.

The depth of colour is proportional to the concentration of the compound being measured and the amount of light absorbed is proportional to the intensity of colour.

SPECTROPHOTOMETRY

The spectrophotometry was invented by Arnold J Beckham and his colleagues in 1940.

It measures the wavelength of light reflected from a sample object or the amount of light that is absorbed by the sample object with variable spectrum like ultraviolet or IR.

Principle

- The instrument operates by passing a beam of light through a sample and measuring the intensity of light reaching a detector.
- Beer Lambert law: It states that there is a linear relationship between the absorbance and the concentration of the sample. Spectrophotometer measures absorbance, transmittance and concentration.
- $a = \epsilon l c$

  where a = absorbance ϵ = molar absorptivity
         l = length of solution c = concentration

Requirements

- **Spectrophotometer:** Producing light of the selected colour
- **Photometer:** Measuring the intensity of light
- **Galvanometer:** Display device

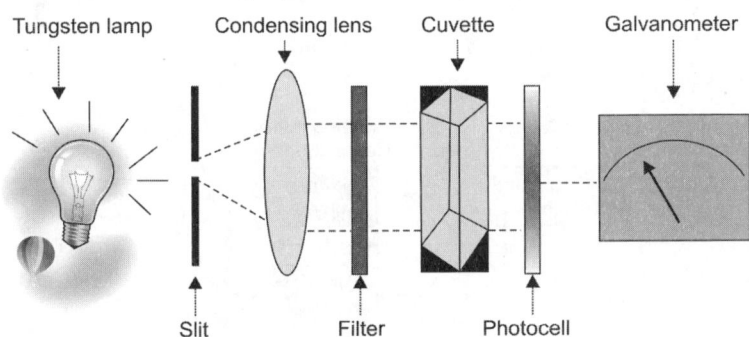

Fig. 8.4: Principle of spectrophotometry

Types of Spectrophotometry

- Single beamed spectrophotometer
- Double beamed spectrophotometer

Single Beamed Spectrophotometer

Procedure

- The instrument is composed of light source, wavelength selector, sample comparator and a detector.
- The spectrum of light is split into its component colours with the help of a wavelength selector and a narrow band spectrum is selected.
- A monochromatic prism is used as a light filter.
- The selected light passes into the sample compartment, then into detector.
- The transmitted light is measured and absorbance is determined.

Double Beamed Spectrophotometer

Procedure

- In addition to the single beamed spectrophotometer, the double beamed spectrophotometer consists of a chopper

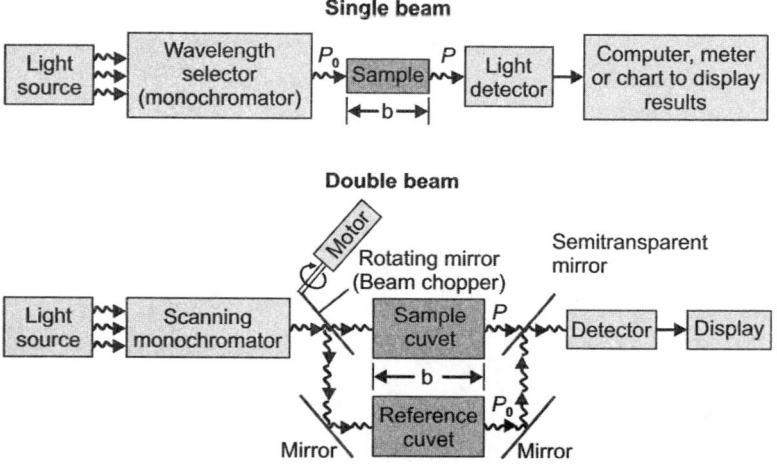

Fig. 8.5: Types of spectrophotometry

motor which deflects the light beam through a reference cell and the sample cell.

- The deflection of light is done many times and the average ratio between the two readings gives the transmittance.
- The double beam spectrophotometer has an advantage that reference reading and sample reading can take place at the same time.

Uses

- To measure the concentration
- Detect impurities
- Detection of functional group
- Molecular weight determination
- Structure elucidation of organic compounds
- Chemical kinetics.

BIBLIOGRAPHY

1. A. Hazra, N. Rege, Practical Pharmacology for Undergraduate Medical Students, New Delhi, Wiley Publishing House, 2014.

Experimental Evaluation

Before the drugs are used in human beings, it is important to study their effects on experimental animals. This gives information about their safety and efficacy. The disease condition is induced in experimental animals by various methods. These are called the animal models for drug screening. Multiple potential molecules are first screened in these models and those found to be safe and effective are later on studied in human volunteers (phase 1 clinical trial). Details are discussed in Chapter 11.

Introduction

Epilepsy is a common neurological disorder characterized by recurrent, unprovoked convulsions. It is largely seen in patients who are less than 20 years of age with increased frequency in old age. Majority of the patients are treated with various anti-epileptic drugs. But there exists a small population of patients who show poor or inadequate response to the AEDs. Therefore, there is a need to develop more effective drugs to reduce the seizure frequency in drug resistant patients so that they have a better safety profile with least side effects.

EVALUATION OF ANTICONVULSANTS

1. **Electrical-induced convulsions**
   - Threshold method
   - Maximum electroshock seizure (MES)
   - Focal stimulation (kindling)

2. **Chemical-induced convulsions**
   - Pentylenetetrazole induced (metrazole/PTZ)
   - INH induced
   - Picrotoxin induced
   - Bicuculine
   - Strychnine induced
   - Penicillin induced
3. **Focal lesion:** Topical application of metal cream/chemicals
4. **Models for status epilepticus**
   - Pilocarpine induced
   - Lithium and pilocarpine induced
5. **Genetic model for epilepsy**

ELECTRICALLY-INDUCED CONVULSIONS

Seizure can be induced in experimental animals by electric stimulation of certain areas of brain. Electric stimulation can be done by corneal/ear electrode by electroconvulsiometer. This can also be done by implanting the electrode in the brain. Efficacy of drug then tested as an anticonvulsant if it blocks the various phases of convulsions.

Threshold Method

Principle

In this method effect of anticonvulsant drug seizure threshold is seen

Procedure

Experimental animal is mice. Animals are divided in control and test group. Test group will receive drug under evaluation while control group will receive normal saline only.

Group	Drug
Test	Drug under evaluation
Positive Control	Standard drug
Negative control	Normal saline/placebo

Electric current is applied with the help of ear/corneal electrode by using electroconvulsiometer. The current is applied with the frequency of 50–60/sec for 0.2 sec.

Parameter for Observation

Current required for inducing tonic limb extension is determined (threshold).

In control group it is 6–9 mA.

Conclusion

Drug is said to be effective if it abolishes the tonic extensor phase and reduces the threshold current by 20%.

> **Note:** Daily administration of current is done. One should not repeat the shock on same day as seizure threshold is increased in post-ictal phase. This will give false result.

Maximal Electroshock Seizure

Principle

In this method the electric current with supramaximal strength is delivered for inducing convulsion. The current strength is 2–5 times higher than the required for testing seizure threshold.

Procedure

The experimental animals, i.e. Swiss albino mice/Wistar rat is divided in test and control groups. Electric current is delivered with corneal/ear electrode.

Electric current can be delivered by two methods. Constant voltage/constant current. If by constant current, in rat—50 mA with the frequency of 50–60/sec for 0.2 sec. In mice it is 150 mA with the frequency of 50–60/sec for 0.2 sec.

With constant voltage 750 V in rat and 250 V in mice.

Conclusion

The drug is considered effective anticonvulsant if it abolishes tonic hind limb extension. Drugs clearing this test are effective against GTCC. Drugs for petit mal will not be able to clear this test.

Various stages of convulsions seen in the animal during this experiment

1. Tonic flexion
2. Tonic extension

3. Clonicgerks
4. Stupor
5. Recovery/death

Kindled Rat Seizure Model

Principle

Repeated stimulation of certain areas of brain by sub-convulsive electric stimulation can induce convulsion in experimental animals.

This is called kindling. Initially there is local after discharge followed by spread of electrical current and later this results into convulsions. Strength of electric current is decided by threshold for convulsion.

Procedure

Experimental animal is either rat/mice. An electrode is placed in the right amygdala/neocortex. After a period of one week (in post-operative period seizure threshold is reduced), the sub-convulsive strength of current is used to stimulate the brain daily (400–500 μA for 1 sec with the frequency of 50–60/sec).

Various Stages of Convulsion

1. Immobility and eye closure
2. Fascial clonus and head nodding
3. Fascial clonus, head nodding and forelimb clonus
4. Rearing
5. Loss of balance with GTCC

Rat is said to be kindled when class 5 seizures has developed.

Advantage: By this method efficacy of drug on patho-physiology of disease/epileptogenesis and efficacy against epilepsy is studied.

Disadvantage: Not able to find out the mechanism of action.

CHEMICAL-INDUCED SEIZURE

In this method the various chemicals as mentioned above are used to induce convulsions (chemoconvulsants).

These chemoconvulsants are administered systemically to produce the convulsions. Some of the examples are pentylene tetrazole/metrazole, strychnine, picrotoxine, isoniazide, bicuculline.

Pentylene tetrazole (PTZ)/Metrazole-induced Convulsions

Principle

PTZ is GABA inhibitory. GABA is inhibitory neurotransmitter, hence parenteral administration of PTZ can cause GTCC in experimental animals.

Clinical Significance

1. Used for screening of drug effective in petit mal epilepsy.
2. Anxiolytic drugs like benzodiazepines have shown anticonvulsant effect in this test.
3. For evaluation of centrally acting skeletal muscle relaxant, this test is recommended.

Procedure

Experimental animal is Wistar rat/Swiss albino mice. Each group should contain 10–12 animals. They are divided in two groups—test and control. PTZ is administered by sc/ip/orally.

Type of convulsion seen after PTZ administration is initially generalised asynchronised followed by GTCC.

Observation

1. Development of tonic clonic convulsions
2. Time taken for onset of convulsions

Note: Minimum 80–90% of animals in control group should show convulsions.

Result

Test group: Number of animals protected
From that calculate ED50

Strychnine-induced Convulsions

Principle

Strychnine antagonises the action of glycine. Glycine is the inhibitory neurotransmitter for motor and interneurons at spinal cord.

Procedure

- Experimental animal is Swiss albino mice. They are divided into three groups.
- Test, control and standard. In standard group all animal receive diazepam (5 mg/kg).
- Strychnine is administered ip in the dose of 2 mg/kg before giving the test and standard drug.

Observations

Animals are observed for development of convulsions.

Various other chemicals can be used for induction of convulsions and these are:

Bicuculin: $GABA_A$ antagonist—2.7 mg/kg/sc in mice
Picrotoxine: $GABA_A$ antagonist—3.5 mgm/kg/sc
Isoniazide: GABA synthesis inhibitors—300 mgm/kg/sc

SEIZURES-INDUCED BY FOCAL LESION

Cortically Implanted Metals

Principle

Focal lesions can be induced by local application of metal like alumina cream (aluminium hydroxide), cobalt and tungstic acid to the cerebral cortex. Also it can be induced by injection of metals like iron. This lesion can cause development of simple partial seizures. Efficacy of the drugs can be tested in simple partial seizures by this model.

Procedure

Experimental animal is monkey. Neocortex of brain is exposed by surgical method. Aluminium hydroxide gel is injected in the neocortex. It takes 1–2 months after injection and seizures persist for several years. Initially partial followed by generalised tonic clonic seizures.

Systemically focal epileptogenesis: Can be done by radiation to cerebrum.

MODELS FOR STATUS EPILEPTICUS

Various animal models are available to study the efficacy of drugs in status epilepticus.

1. **Pilocarpine-induced status epilepticus:** Experimental animal is rat. Pilocarpine is given in the dose 300–400 mgm/kg by ip route. This induces status epilepticus in experimental animal.
2. **Pilocarpine and lithium-induced status epilepticus:** Experimental animal is rat. Pilocarpine is given in the dose 30–40 mgm/kg and lithium is given in the dose of 3 meq/kg by ip route 24 hours before pilocarpine. This induces status epilepticus in experimental animal.

Genetic Models for Epilepsy

Experimental animals are photosensitive baboons. Convulsions are induced by intermittent flashes of light in the frequency of 25 flashes/second.

EVALUATION OF ANTI-DEPRESSANTS

Introduction

Depression is a common mental disorder that presents with low mood, anhedonia, low self-worth, disturbed sleep and poor concentration, suicidal thoughts and attempts. It may adversely affect cognition or psychomotor function. Depression is the 4th leading cause of global burden of disease. The existing animal models should be modified to detect compounds acting on them as new targets are being developed:
• Despair swim test
• Tail suspension test
• Learned helplessness
• Compulsory gnawing test
• Apo morphine-induced hypothermia
• Reserpine-induced hypothermia
• Serotonin syndrome in rat
• Tetrabenazine antagonism in mice

1. Despair Swim Test

Procedure

Experimental animal is male Sprague dawley rat. One day prior animals are housed in propylene cage with access to adequate water and food. Next day animals are subjected to forced swimming individually in a vertical glass cylinder. Dimensions of cylinder are height —40 cm, width —18 cm, height of water column—15 cm and temperature of water—25°C.

Observations

1. Animals start swimming vigorously in the beginning.
2. After a period of 2–3 minutes swimming period reduces and animal tries to escape by climbing all the wall of cylinder.
3. Followed by that animal remains immobilised for majority of the period
4. Immobility—this includes hunched out upright posture with only nose on surface.

Parameter for Observation

Period of immobility

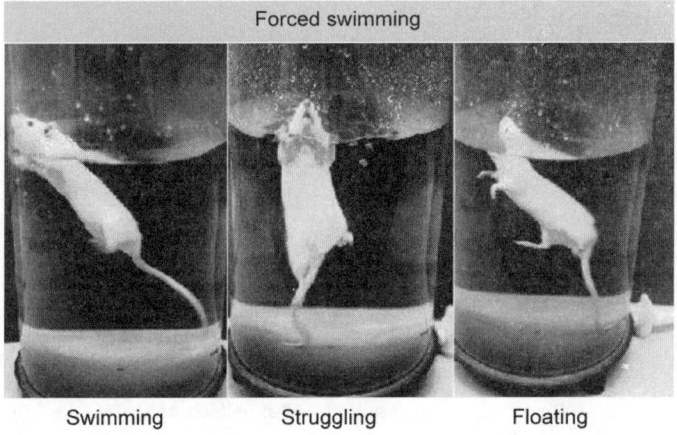

Fig. 9.1: Forced swim test

Conclusion

Antidepressant drugs reduce the period of immobility significantly.

2. Tail Suspension Test

Principle

When animal is exposed to unavoidable and inescapable stress, there is characteristic immobile posture change seen in the animal. This reflects the major manifestation of depression in the human. Potential antidepressant drug will reduce this characteristic behaviour.

Procedure

Experimental animal: Mice. These group of animals are divided into test and control. Test group will receive drug under evaluation by ip/oral route. Animals are suspended in an inverted position by applying the adhesive tape at 1 cm away from tip of the tail. Animals are suspended at the edge of table.

Observation

Animals will hang passively and later on completely motionless. Period of immobility for 60 sec is considered significant.

Conclusion

Potential antidepressant will reduce the period of immobility.

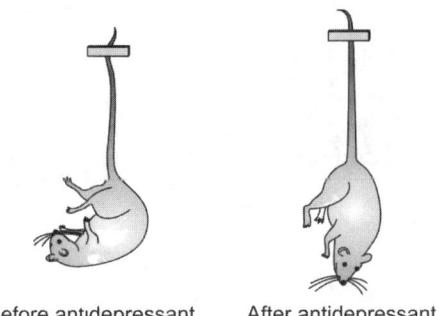

Before antidepressant   After antidepressant

Fig. 9.2: Tail suspension test

3. Compulsory Gnawing Test in Mice

Principle

Apomorphine is the dopamine agonist. Its administration in human causes vomiting in human because of action on D2 receptors, experimental animal causes compulsory gnawing, stereotyped behaviour, climbing and hypothermia. Antidepressant drugs will block the compulsory gnawing.

Procedure

Experimental animals: Mice. They are divided into control and test group. Animals are kept into the cages having upward corrugation paper at the base. Injection apomorpheine 16 mgm/kg/sc is given to the animals.

Observation

Animal will start biting the corrugated paper. If drug has anti-depressant effect, it will reduce the biting/gnawing.

Apomorphine-induced Hypothermia

Apomorphine injection will induce hypothermia in the experimental animal (mice). This is measured by rectal thermometer. It is measured at the interval of 10, 20 and 30 minutes.

Conclusion

Antidepressant will block the apomorphine-induced hypothermia.

Significance

Neuroleptic will block climbing and stereotyped behaviour but not hypothermia.

Reserpine-induced Hypothermia

Experimental animals: Mice.

Procedure

Reserpine is injected in the dose of 2.5–5 mgm/kg by sc route. This will cause ptosis, catalepsy and hypothermia in mice. Potential antidepressant will cause reversal of this effect.

Learned Helplessness in Rats

Experimental animal: Sprague-Dawley rat

Principle

Exposing the animals to inescapable and unavoidable electric shocks in a situation leads to failing to escape shock in a different situation when escape is possible.

Procedure

The animals are exposed to electric shock via a grid floor for an hour; 10 sec shock/min. A platform is inserted through one side of the wall to allow a jump-up escape response which is not made available during training. The animal is treated and tested for jump up escape response. A drug is considered to be effective if the learned helplessness is reduced and the number of failures to escape is decreased.

EVALUATION OF ANTIPSYCHOTIC AGENTS

Drugs used for treatment of schizophrenia are called antipsychotics. Schizophrenia also called split mind is a type of psychoses. It is a severe psychiatric illness and characterised by serious distortion of thought, behaviour and capacity to recognize reality and of perception (delusions and hallucinations).

Pathophysiology of Schizophrenia

Dopamine theory of schizophrenia: Various antipsychotics act by blockade of dopaminergic projections in the limbic system and in mesocortical areas. This along with the observation that drugs which increase DA activity, i.e. amphetamines, levodopa, bromocriptine induce or exacerbate schizophrenia. Hence dopamine overactivity in limbic area is responsible for the condition.

Various Antipsychotic Drugs

- *Typical/first generation*: Chlorpromazine, haloperidol
- *Atypical/second generation*: Newer drugs like clozapine, olanzapine

  Various models and methods for evaluation of antipsychotics
  1. Catalepsy in rodents
  2. Innate behaviour of golden hamster
  3. Antagonism of amphetamine induced stereotyped behaviour
  4. Inhibition of jumping in mice
  5. Apomorphine climbing in mice

Catalepsy in Rodents

Principle

Catalepsy means inability of animal to correct the externally imposed posture for a long period of time. It manifests as immobility, body stiffness and inability to initiate the movements. This mimics the extrapyramidal effects of antipsychotics. This is because of inhibition of niagrostriatal dopaminergic tract. This model is used to test the extrapyramidal effects of potential antipsychotics.

Procedure

Experimental animals are male Wistar rats. They are divided into test and control group.

Animals are tested for catalepsy score. This is measured by keeping the front both paws on the column with height of 3 cm and 9 cm. It is scored as inability of the animal to correct the posture.

Catalepsy score	Observation	Time
Score 1	Inability to correct the position from the height of 3 cm for 10 sec.	Score is tested at the gap of 30 min for 2 hours
Score 2	Inability to correct the position from the height of 9 cm for 10 sec.	Score is tested at the gap of 30 min for 2 hours.

Result

Higher the score, more chances of it to cause the EPS in human.

Innate Behaviour in Golden Hamster

Principle

Male golden hamster has aggressive behaviour. Neuroleptic drugs have taming/calming effect on their behaviour. This can be used in the screening of neuroleptic drugs.

Procedure

Male golden hamsters are divided into two groups—control and test.

Before experiment 20–25 animals are caged together for 15 days, this is for increasing their aggressive behaviour. Later on the animals are housed singly in the glass cylinder with capacity of 2–3 litres. Animals are tested for their aggressive behaviour by punching with the forceps. Three responses are seen and which include turning on back, vocalising and biting the forceps in defensive action. Only such animals are selected.

Observations

In test group the drug under evaluation is given by sc/ip route. In control group the animal will receive standard drug/vehicle like NS. Animal is observed for aggressive behaviour by stimulating with forceps. The compound is tested/compared with standard drug for taming effect. This is indicated by reduction in the aggressive behaviour.

Neuroleptic width

Neuroleptic will affect the motor tone in higher doses. Neuroleptic width is the ratio between ED50 for taming effect and ED50 for motor function. It is commonly between 1.5 and 1.30.

Effect on motor function is tested by ability to maintain posture on inclined plane with the angle of 20°.

Advantages

1. This differentiates between neuroleptic and sedative hypnotic.
2. This test is very simple and does not require any training.

Inhibition of Jumping in Mice

Principle

Neuroleptic drugs have inhibitory effect on dopaminergic neurones. While amphetamine (indirectly acting sympathomimetic) and levodopa (dopamine facilitator) increase dopamine effect. If both these drugs dopamine stimulators are given together, they will cause hyperdopaminergic effects. This will induce excessive jumping in the mice and will be blocked by neuroleptics.

Antagonism of Amphetamine-induced Stereotyped Behaviour

Experimental animal: Adult white leghorn chicken

Procedure

The animal is held with both the hands and placed on its back for a minute. Cataleptic numbness occurs immediately. This state can remain for an hour. The cataleptic rigor can be interrupted by noise or fast movements. The animals are screened for their cataleptic behaviour. The same animal is used as control and test. Test is considered positive if the cataleptic rigor does not occur after the treatment or is interrupted within a minute.

Criteria for positive response: Suppression of cataleptic phenomenon.

Apomorphine-induced Hyperthermia in Mice

Experimental animal: NMRI mice

Procedure

Test drugs are given orally. Rectal temperature of each mouse is measured by an electronic thermometer prior to giving the test drug, at 10, 20 and 30 minutes. Compounds with marked noradrenergic or dopaminergic components are active against apomorphine-induced hypothermia but not the ones which act via serotonergic receptors.

Apomorphine Climbing in Mice

Experimental animal: Mice

Procedure

The animals are treated with intraperitoneal injections of test or vehicle compound, after which they are given subcutaneous injections of apomorphine. A typical climbing behaviour starting with rearing and then leading to full climbing activity is seen when mice are treated with apomorphine and it is noted at 10, 20 and 30 minutes of apomorphine injection.

Scoring

0 = All the four paws of the animal are on the floor
1 = Forefeet of the animal holding the vertical bars
2 = Forefeet holding the vertical bars

EXPERIMENTAL EVALUATION OF LOCAL ANAESTHETICS

Local anaesthetics (LA) are drugs which upon local application or local injection cause reversible loss of sensory perception, especially of pain, in a restricted area of the body.

Classification

Injectable anaesthetics

Low potency, short duration
• Procaine, chloroprocaine

Intermediate potency and duration
• Lidocaine (lignocaine)

High potency, long duration
• Tetracaine, bupivacaine
• Ropivacaine, dibucaine

Surface anaesthetics

• Cocaine, lidocaine, tetracaine
• Benzocaine, oxethazaine

1. Infiltration anaesthesia in guinea pig
2. Surface anaesthesia/topical anaesthesia in rabbit
   • Loss of blinking reflex
   • Abolition of sneezing
3. Conduction block
   • Sciatic nerve block in rat/frog
   • Conduction block in mouse tail
4. Epidural anaesthesia in guinea pig
5. Spinal anaesthesia in rat
   Various techniques used for evaluation of LA.

• **Surface anaesthesia:** In this method local anaesthetic drug is applied topically to the mucous membranes and abraded skin. Only superficial layer is anaesthetised, e.g. lignocaine spray in the throat acts in 2–5 min and lasts for 30–45 min. Short procedures like removal of foreign body from cornea, proctoscopy, etc.

• **Infiltration anaesthesia:** In this technique dilute solution of local anaesthetic is infiltrated under the skin over the operative field which blocks sensory nerve endings. Onset of action is rapid but duration is shorter than nerve block. Various minor operations done under it are incisions, excisions, hydrocele, herniorrhaphy.

- **Conduction block:** The local anaesthetic is infiltrated around nerve trunks so that the area distal to the injection is anaesthetised and paralysed.
- **Field block:** It is produced by injecting the local anaesthetic subcutaneously in a manner that all nerves coming to a particular field are blocked, e.g. herniorrhaphy, appendicectomy.
- **Spinal anaesthesia:** In this technique the local anaesthetic solution is injected in the subarachnoid space between L2–3 and L3–4 space, i.e. below the lower end of spinal cord. Lower abdomen and hindlimbs are anaesthetised and paralysed. Duration of anaesthesia depends upon the drug, e.g. lignocaine—45 mins and bupivacaine 2 hours.

    Various surgical procedures done under it are:
    - Gynaecological procedures like hysterectomy, caesarean section
    - Lower abdominal procedures like appendicectomy

    Complications of spinal anaesthesia
    - Spinal hypotension
    - Spinal headache
    - Meningitis
    - Respiratory paralysis
- **Epidural anaesthesia:** Diluted solution of LA is injected in the epidural space. It has advantage over epidural of less chances of hypotension.

EXPERIMENTS FOR EVALUATION OF ANAESTHETICS

Surface Anaesthesia

Animal: Corneal anaesthesia in rabbits
Human volunteers: Taste sensation and ethyl chloride spray

Corneal Anaesthesia in Rabbits

Requirements

Experimental animal: Rabbit (with trimmed eyelashes)
Equipment: Rabbit holder, cotton wick
Drugs: Local anaesthetic solution
Blinking reflex: Closure of eyelid when cornea is touched with cotton wick

Procedure

1. Place the rabbit in rabbit holder
2. Check the active blinking reflex before adding drug in eye
3. Add 2–3 drops of test drug in eye
4. Check the reflex post drug
   Result: Loss of blinking reflex indicate LA action

Infiltration Anaesthesia in Guinea Pig

Requirements

Experimental animal: Guinea pig with circular fashioned shaved area on both side of back

   Drugs: LA and normal saline
   Syringe and needle

Procedure

1. Inject 0.2 ml of LA solution on one side of back and 0.2 ml of NS on the other side of back (control).
2. Test the pin prick sensation on both sides.
3. Loss of response to pin prick, indicate local anaesthetic action.

LA Evaluation in Human Volunteers

Requirement

• Healthy human volunteer with written inform consent
• Concentrated solution of glucose
• LA solution

Procedure

1. Add a drop of concentrated glucose solution on the middle of tongue.
2. Ask for sweet taste sensation
3. Followed by that add a drop of LA solution and again glucose drop
4. Loss of taste indicates LA action

Abolition of Sneezing in Rabbit

Experimental animal: New Zealand albino rabbit

Procedure

One of the nostrils acts as control. Fine lead pencil tip is used to stimulate the mucosa. Reflex is tested before and after application of drug.

Parameter for observation

Loss of sneezing reflex on stimulating the nasal mucosa.

Conduction Block

Sciatic Nerve Block in Rat

Experimental animal: Male Wistar rat

Procedure

Sciatic nerve is blocked by injection of diluted solution of drug under evaluation at the junction of bicep femoris and gluteus maximus.

Parameter for evaluation: Foot drop (walking behaviour) and proximity of the digits of the leg.

Conduction Block in Mouse Tail

Experimental animal: Swiss albino mice

Procedure

Test and control drug is injected in the tail.

Parameter for observation: Withdrawal of tail on exposure to radiant heat by analgesiometer.

Epidural Anaesthesia in Guinea Pig

Experimental animal: Guinea pig

Procedure

Under anaesthesia epidural catheter is inserted in the epidural space (Lumbosacral). The catheter is secured. Drug under evaluation is injected in the catheter. Bilateral sensory and motor loss indicate local anaesthetic activity.

EXPERIMENTAL EVALUATION OF SEDATIVE AND HYPNOTIC DRUGS

Sedative: A drug that subdues excitement and calms the subject without inducing sleep, though drowsiness may be produced.

Hypnotic: A drug that induces and/or maintains sleep, similar to normal arousable sleep.

Drugs Used

- Barbiturates
- Benzodiazepines
- Nonbenzodiazepine hypnotics

    Various experimental methods used are:
    - Fall time method: Rota rod apparatus and inclined plane.
    - Cooke's pole climbing (conditioned avoidance response)
    - Actophotometer
    - Taming effect in animal
    - Aggregation toxicity

ROTAROD APPARATUS

Principle

Benzodiazepines (diazepam) are the most popular sedative and hypnotic agents. These drugs have taming/calming effect together with muscle relaxant action. This effect can be easily studied in animals by using rotarod/inclined plane.

Parameter for observation: The difference in the fall off time from the rotating rod between the control and test groups.

Requirements

Experimental animals used: Mice
Drugs: Normal saline (NS), drug under evaluation (test)
Equipment: Rotarod

Procedure

1. Weigh the animals and number them
2. Divide them in control (A) and test (B) group (minimum 4 in each group)
3. Turn on rotarod. Select the appropriate speed (12 revolution/min.)
4. Place the animal one by one on the rotating rod. Note down the 'fall of time' for each animal. (Generally normal mouse falls off within 3–5 min.)

5. Administered the test drug and control (NS) by subcutaneous/oral route.
6. Post-treatment again measure the score (no. of fall and duration of performance) in all animals.

Results

Increase number of falls and reduce period of performance suggest that the drug has either CNS depressant/skeletal muscle relaxant property.

Conditioned Avoidance Response

Aim

Differentiate between minor and major tranquillizers.

Minor tranquillizers: These are most commonly used drugs in psychopharmacology and have CNS depressant and skeletal muscle relaxant property, e.g. benzodiazepines.

Major tranquillizers: These are the CNS depressant drugs with no skeletal muscle relaxant action and less commonly used, e.g. antipsychotics.

Experimental animals: Trained rats

Drugs: Normal saline and test drug

Equipments: Cook's pole climbing apparatus

Conditioned response: Animal will respond to both shock and buzzer

Unconditioned response: Response to buzzer will be lost

Apparatus: It includes a wooden box with iron grill at the bottom and hanging wooden pole from the roof.

Training: Animals are subjected to the training as below:
1. Animal is kept in the apparatus
2. Grill of apparatus connected to electric circuit
3. To avoid shock, animal will climb on the rod
4. Now the buzzer is put on followed by shock
5. Next time animal will be conditioned to buzzer and will climb before shock

Result

Drugs	Avoidance response	
	Unconditioned	Conditioned
Normal saline	Present	Present
Minor tranquilizer	Absent	Absent
Major tranquilizer	Present	Absent

Taming Effect in Animal

Principle

When one animal is exposed to the other which is its prey, the first animal will show a peculiar behaviour. Tranquillizer will tame it and there will be change of behaviour.

Procedure

1. Exposure of cat to the rat will show a hostile behaviour.
2. After administration of minor tranquillizer, cat will be silent and withdrawn.

EVALUATION OF ANTIHYPERTENSIVE DRUG

Introduction

Hypertension is the most common cardiovascular disorder; defined as a sustained increase in the blood pressure $\geq 140/90$ mmHg. The animal models of hypertension share many features which are common to human hypertension. Many of these models have been developed by utilizing the etiological factors that are presumed to be responsible for hypertension.

Evaluation of Antihypertensive Drugs

1. Acute renal hypertension in rats (2K1C)—Goldblatt method
2. Chronic renal hypertension in rats (1K1C)
3. Fructose fed hypertension
4. DOCA salt-induced hypertension in rats
5. Genetic hypertension in rats
6. Spontaneous hypertension in rats

Acute Renal Hypertension in Rats (2K1C) Goldblatt Method

Experimental animal: Sprague-Dawley Rat

Principle

Renal ischemia increases blood pressure in rat by activating RAAS.

Procedure

The animal is anaesthetized with hexobarbital. Left kidney and hilum is exposed. Renal artery is occluded (left) with PVC coated clip for 4 hours, followed by that the clamp is reopened. This increased blood pressure after reopening is reduced by the test compound.

Chronic Renal Hypertension in Rats (1K1C)

Experimental animal: Rat

Principle

Constriction of renal artery on one side and the contralateral kidney is removed. Marked increase in blood pressure takes place within a few hours. Because of non-functioning of both the kidneys there is salt water retention.

Procedure

The animal is anaesthetized with pentobarbitone. Renal artery is identified and usher silver clip is applied. Contralateral kidney is removed. The rats are observed for one and a half months after clipping. Test and control drugs are administered during this period.

Salt Sensitive Dahl Rats

Experimental animal: Sprague-Dawley rat

Principle

Genetically salt sensitive rats are fed on high salt diet. This results in development of fatal and severe hypertension.

Procedure

The animals are fed on salt by replacing drinking water with 8% NaCl. Regular diet is mixed with salt and fed to the animals.

Blood pressure starts to rise after 1 week and persistently increased up to 4 weeks. Then these animals are divided into the control and test one for the evaluation of antihypertensive drug almost for 1 month.

DOCA and Salt-induced Hypertension in Rats

Experimental animal: Male Sprague-Dawley rat

Principle

DOCA (de-oxy corticosterone acetate) which is a mineralo-corticoid increases salt and water retention. The hypertensive effect is further enhanced by salt loading and unilateral nephrectomy.

Procedure

The animals undergo nephrectomy under general anaesthesia. DOCA is given 20 mgm/kg/sc twice a week for 4 weeks. Salt loading is done by replacing drinking water with 1% NaCl. Hypertension develops after 1 week. Blood pressure start rising from 1 week and reaches to 160–180 mmHg by 4 weeks. These animals are divided into test and control group for evaluation of antihypertensive drugs.

Fructose-induced Hypertension in Rat

Experimental animal: Wistar rat

Principle

Fructose which is a carbohydrate induces insulin resistance and hypertension.

Procedure

Fructose is fed to the animals by replacing drinking water with 10% fructose solution. Hypertension develops within 6 weeks. These animals are divided into test and control groups for evaluation of antihypertensive drugs.

Neurogenic Model

Experimental animal: Dog

Principle

Neurogenic control of blood pressure is done by carotid sinus and aortic arch through VMC and vagus nerve. Sectioning of them can cause persistent rise in blood pressure.

Procedure

Experimental animal is adult dog. Dog is anaesthetised and femoral vein is cannulated for drug administration and blood pressure is measured by femoral artery. Bilateral vagotomy is done and nerve supply to carotid sinus is blocked. A period of 30 min is given to establish the equilibrium. Followed by that the drug is administered as intravenous bolus.

Spontaneously Hypertensive Rats

Experimental animal: Spontaneously hypertensive rats (SHR)

Principle

The strain is known as Wistar Kyoto rats (WKY) or Okamoto-Aoki- SHR rats. The genetically sensitive rat strain is developed by mating Wistar male (spontaneously hypertensive) with a female rat (slightly high blood pressure). Repeated breeding results into development of strain with high systolic blood pressure up to 200 mmHg). Various strains are develop, very popular stroke prone strain SHR.

EVALUATION OF ANTI-ARRHYTHMIC DRUGS

Introduction

An arrhythmia is a disorder of the heart rate or heart rhythm. The heart can beat too fast, too slow or irregularly. Prevalence of arrhythmia in India: >20 million.

The screening of anti-arrhythmics is done by two different methods:

In vitro Models

• Lagendroff technique

In vivo Models

• Animal models for atrial arrhythmias

- Aconitine-induced atrial arrhythmias
- Acetylcholine induced
- Crush-cum-electrical stimulation
- Animal models for ventricular arrhythmias (ABCDE + VO)
  - Aconitine induced
  - Barium chloride
  - Calcium chloride induced
  - Digoxine induced
  - Epinephrine induced
  - Veratrum induced
  - Occlusion of coronary artery

In vivo methods can be classified as:
- Chemically-induced arrhythmia—
  - Aconitine, digoxine, adrenaline, etc. induced
- Electrically-induced arrhythmia
- Mechanically-induced arrhythmia
- Exercise-induced arrhythmia

Normal Sinus Rhythm
SA node fibres at 60–100 beats/sec → Spreads through atria → Enters the AV node (delay of 0.15 sec) → Propagates through His-Purkinje system → Depolarizes ventricles beginning from endocardial surface of apex to epicardial surface of base →

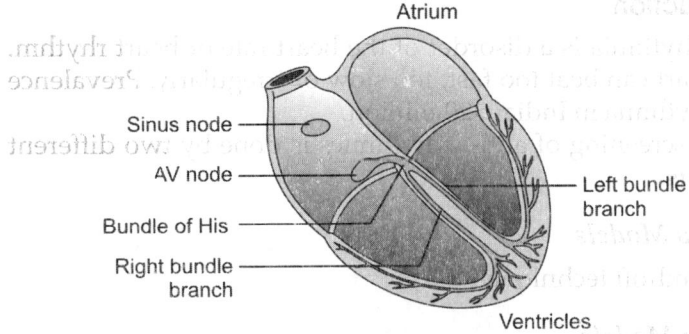

Fig. 9.3: Anatomy of heart

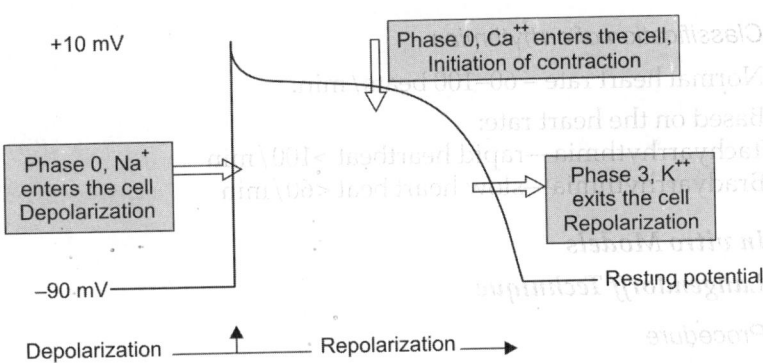

Fig. 9.4: Monophasic action potential (cardiac muscles cell)

Cardiac Arrhythmia

It is defined as deviation from normal of any of the following: Origin/conduction/rhythm/rate. Mainly occurs in patients who have acute MI, taking digitalis or in anaesthetized patients.

Normal ECG

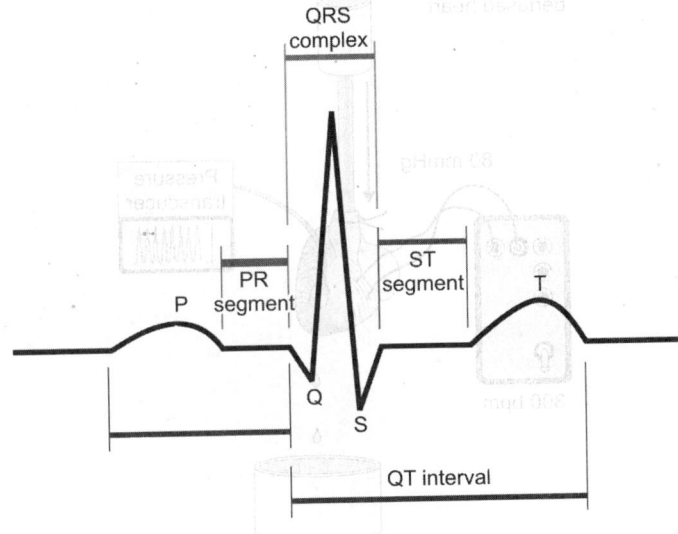

Fig. 9.5

Classification of arrhythmias

Normal heart rate – 60–100 beats/min.

Based on the heart rate:
Tachyarrhythmia—rapid heartbeat >100/min
Bradyarrhythmia—slow heart beat <60/min

In vitro Models
Langendorff Technique

Procedure

Experimental animal: Guinea pig (300–500)

Procedure

Animal sacrificed (stunning) → heart is removed → placed in Ringer's solution (37°C) → aorta is located, cut and cannulated with Ringer's solution (perfused at 40 mmHg) → Ligature is placed around LAD ligature → test/std/control— administered → occluded for 10 minutes → reperfusion is done → with ECG pulsatile stimulation is done → induction of arrhythmia → heart rate and contractile force—measured.

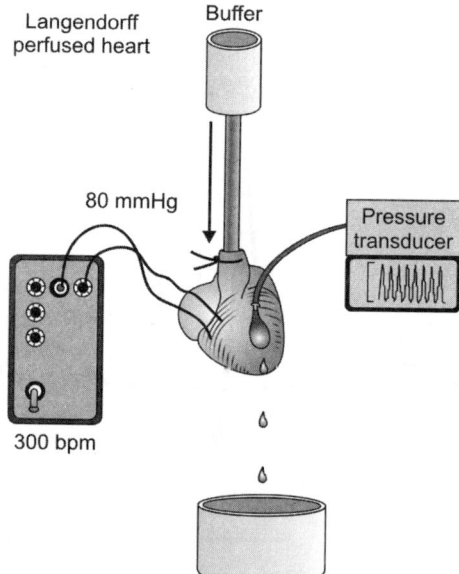

Fig. 9.6: Langendorff technique

Parameter for observation

1. Heart rate measured by chronometer
2. Contractile force is measured by force transducer
3. Incidence and duration of ventricular fibrillation or ventricular tachycardia is recorded in the control as well as test group.

In vivo **Methods**

Aconitine-induced Atrial Arrhythmias

Experimental animal: Dog

Procedure

Animals are selected → anaesthetized with urathene 1.25 g/kg → test/std/control drug is administered → aconitine (5 µg/kg dissolved in 0.1N HNO_3) (administered through saphenous vein) → ECG is recorded (lead II).

Evaluation

The anti-arrhythmic effect of the test compound is measured by the amount of aconitine/100 gm animal (infusion duration), required to precipitate.

Ventricular extra systoles, ventricular tachycardia, ventricular fibrillation and death.

Acetylcholine-induced Atrial Arrhythmias

Experimental animal: New Zealand white rabbits

Procedure

Animals are sacrificed and heart is removed. The atria is dissected out and kept in Ringer's solution. An electrode is attached to the atria and fibrillation is produced with acetylcholine and the tracings are recorder on a kymograph. Test compound is effective if fibrillation disappears immediately or by 5 minutes following test drug into the organ bath.

Crush-cum-electrical Stimulation

Experimental animal: Dogs (8–12 kg)

Procedure

Dog is anaesthetized with sodium pentobarbital (35 mg/kg) → artificial respiration is given by Harvard respiratory pump → BP is monitored and body temperature is maintained by thermal blanket → chest cavity is opened and → heart suspended in pericardial cradle → SA node is crushed → Ag-AgCl electrode embedded in a teflon disc—sutured on left ventricle for electric impulse → Test drug/std/control is given by femoral artery → constant current for 400 ms is applied through electrode.

Evaluation

ECG (Lead II) — monitored and VFT is measured (minimal current intensity required to induce sustained ventricular fibrillation)

Coronary Artery Occlusion/reperfusion Arrhythmia (mechanical)

Experimental animal: Dog

Principle

Arrhythmias can be induced directly by ischemia and reperfusion. In anaesthetized dogs coronary artery ligation causes ↑ in HR, ↑in heart contractility, ↑in BP and ventricular arrhythmias.

Procedure

Dog is anaesthetized with thiobutobarbital sodium (30 mg/kg) → artificial respiration is given → femoral artery is cannulated and connected to pressure transducer → chest cavity is opened and LAD is exposed→ For occlusion silk suture is placed around LAD → After 45 minutes test/std/control is administered through saphenous vein →After 20 minutes ligature of coronary artery is closed for 90 minutes → Occlusion is released and reperfusion period maintained for 30 minutes. All the parameters are recorded →At the end surviving animals are sacrificed by an overdose of pentobarbital sodium.

EVALUATION OF ANTI-ANGINAL DRUGS

Introduction

Angina pectoris; the primary symptom of ischemic heart disease is caused by transient episodes of myocardial ischemia that are caused due to the imbalance in the myocardial oxygen supply–demand relationship. Obesity, insulin resistance and type II diabetes mellitus are increasing and are an important risk factor for IHD.

In vitro

- Langendorff heart preparation
- Calcium antagonism in rat
- Bovine coronary artery relaxation
- Isolated coronary artery ligation in rat
- Plastic cast techniques in dog

In vivo Animal (Intact Animal)

- Occlusion of coronary artery
  - Coronary artery ligation in rat
  - Coronary artery ligation in dog
  - Microsphere-induced LVF
  - Coronary artery stenosis in dogs
  - Electrical stimulation-induced coronary thrombosis
  - Isoproterenol-induced myocardial necrosis
  - Ischaemic preconditioning

Langendorff Heart Preparation

Experimental animal: Guinea pig heart

Principle

Heart is perfused in a retrograde direction from aorta with oxygenated saline solution which closes the aortic valves, same as in the *in situ* heart during diastole. Parameters observed are coronary flow, contractility and rhythm.

Procedure

The guinea pig is sacrificed by a blow on the head. The heart is isolated along with the aorta and vena cava. It is immediately placed in the doubled wall plexi-glass perfusion apparatus at 37°C. Oxygenated Ringer's solution is used as a perfusion fluid. The parameters measure heart rate—with chronometer, coronary blood flow, force of contraction, potassium levels after treatment within the drug. This method is useful for testing coronary vasodilator drug.

Calcium Antagonism in Rats

Experimental animal: Sprague-Dawley rat.

Principle and Procedure

Continuous electric stimulation of thoracic cord is used to produce tachycardia. The drug is administered through jugular vein and blood pressure is recorded via carotid artery. The potential of the test drug to reduce tachycardia is used as anti-ischaemic property.

Relaxation of Bovine Coronary Artery

Experimental animal: Cow

Procedure

The spiral strips from bovine coronary artery are immersed in oxygenated Krebs solution. The test compound is administered in the solution and the relaxation produced is measured. PGI2 is used as a standard.

Coronary Artery Ligation in Isolated Rat Heart

Experimental animal: Wistar rats

Procedure

Acute ischemia is produced by clamping the left coronary artery. The clip is then opened and changes during reperfusion period are monitored. Parameters like left ventricular pressure, heart rate and coronary flow are measured.

Plastic Casts Techniques in Dogs

Test animal: Dogs, pigs

Procedure

Dogs are anaesthetized with pentobarbital sodium. The animal is maintained on artificial respiration. The chest cavity is opened and the heart is exposed. Cuffs are placed around the coronaries. These plastic materials swell gradually and occlude the lumen in 3–4 weeks.The test drug increases the number and size of inter-arterial collaterals. Plastic casts are used to quantify the collaterals.

In vivo Models

Occlusion of Coronary Artery

Experimental animal: Dog

Principle

Compounds that reduce infarct size are studied using this model. Infarct size is studied after LAD coronary artery occlusion.

Microspheres-induced Acute Ischemia

Experimental animal: Dogs

Procedure

Left ventricular failure is induced by injecting microspheres in left main coronary artery. Drugs are tested on the basis of their improvement in cardiac performance.

Isoproterenol-induced Myocardial Necrosis

Experimental animal: Wistar rat

Procedure

Isoprotenol (synthetic catecholamine) produces cardiac necrosis. Changes in histological, biochemical and hemodynamic diameters are measured.

Stenosis-induced Coronary Thrombosis

Experimental animal: Dogs

Procedure

Thrombosis is induced by producing stenosis in dogs by alterations in the blood flow in the coronaries. The test compound is given intravenously and the cyclic flow variations are compared to pre-treatment values.

EVALUATION OF ANALGESICS

Introduction

Analgesics are the drug which increases pain threshold for pain and reduces/abolishes the pain.

Analgesics are classified as:

1. Opioids/narcotics
2. Non-opioids/non-narcotics

Experimental methods are divided as follows:

1. Animal models for acute pain
2. Animal models for chronic pain
3. Human evaluation/Clinical methods

Animal Models for Acute Pain

Thermal (heat stimulus)

- Hot plate method—Eddy's hot plate
- Tail-flick test—By using radiant heat (analgesiometer)
- Immersion of the tail in warm water
- Immersion of the tail in cold water and ethylene glycol

Electrical stimulus

- Tooth pulp test

Chemical stimulus

- Writhing test
- Rat sigmoid colon model
- Inflammatory uterine pain model

Mechanical stimulus

- Tail clip method (Haffneris method)
- Randall-Selitto test

Animal Models For Chronic Pain

- Neuropathic pain model
- Rat model for bone cancer pain
- Vincristine-induced neuropathy model
- Persistent post-thoracotomy pain model
- Rat model of incisional pain

THERMAL METHOD

Tail-Flick Method

Aim

1. Test the potency of opioid analgesic
2. Discrimination between opioid and non-opioid analgesics

Advantage: Minimum inter-animal variation

Flick response: Application of heat stimulus causes withdrawal of tail by characteristic way.

Tail-flick test—by using radiant heat

Instrument: Analgesiometer

Analgesiometer is raised to bright red heat. Animal is positioned to keep the tail in contact with wire. After a certain time the animal withdraws his tail by sudden and characteristic flick. Time required to do this is considered as reaction time. Reaction time is tested before and after giving analgesic prolongation of reaction time is a measure of analgesic effect.

Alternative to Tail-flick method—immersion of tail in hot water

Procedure: distal part of tail 5 cm is immersed in hot water at 55°C and increase in reaction time after giving analgesic indicates analgesic activity.

Tail-flick method—immersion of tail in cold water and ethylene glycol

Procedure: Distal part of tail 5 cm is immersed in cold water at −10°C and ethylene glycol mixture kept in the test tube and increase in reaction time after giving analgesic indicates analgesic activity.

Eddy's Hot Plate

Procedure: Experimental animals are mice and electrically heated plate with temperature of 55–60°C is used as an equipment.

Parameter for observation: Time taken for jumping, licking and withdrawal of paw. Increase reaction time indicates analgesic activity.

Electrical Stimulus: Tooth Pulp Test/Tail

Procedure: Experimental animal is rabbit. Inj. thiopentone is given in the dose of 15 mg/kg IV and the pulp of central incisors is exposed with dental drill.

Electrode is placed after 30 min. The pulp is stimulated with electric current of 0.2 mA/sec.

Parameter for observation: Licking of tooth

Result: Increase reaction time indicates analgesic activity

Same procedure is applied for tail.

Mechanical method

Haffneris tail clip method: Preferred sites for pressure application are hindpaw and tail. This method is highly sensitive for centrally acting analgesics. Gradual increase in pressure is used than constant pressure application.

Procedure: Experimental animal is mice. Artery clip is applied at the base of tail. There will be characteristic backward movement of head to remove the clip called **squeak response.** Increase reaction time indicates analgesic activity.

Randall-Selitto test: This test is used to detect peripheral analgesic activity.

Principle: Inflammation reduces the pain threshold and thereby increases pain sensitivity. Brewer's yeast is administered subcutaneously for induction of inflammation. Followed by that pressure is applied by specific instrument called Randall-Selitto apparatus.

Procedure: Wistar rats are the experimental animal. Animals are divided into control and test groups. Brewer's yeast 20% suspension in the volume of 0.1 ml is injected subcutaneously in the plantar aspect of hind paw. Pressure is applied with Randall-Selitto after 3 hours.

Parameter for observation: Struggling of animal because of pain. Increase reaction time indicates analgesic activity.

Writing test (chemical stimulus): Intraperitoneal injection of acetic acid elicit a characteristic stretching response (within 3 to 10 min), this is called writhing. Writhing is stretching of anterior abdominal wall with separation of hindlimb. No. of episodes over 10 min periods are recorded before and after giving analgesics. Decreased in no. of stretching episodes suggests analgesic activity.

ANIMAL MODEL FOR CHRONIC PAIN

Neuropathic Pain

Experimental animal: Rat

Procedure: Under halothane anaesthesia the sciatic nerve is isolated. Then a loose knot is tied around it. After a few days animal shows foot drop.

Now animals are divided into control and test group. Analgesic is administered into the test group. Thermal stimulus is applied by a halothane lamp.

Result: Withdrawal reaction is observed in both groups. Increase reaction time indicates analgesic activity of the compound.

Clinical Evaluation Methods

Capsaicin-induced neurogenic inflammation in intact human skin

Procedure: Drug used is capsaicin (1000 μgm / 20 μl). It is applied on the frontal/ventral aspect of the both the forearm in healthy human volunteers.

Parameter for observation: Dermal blood flow is measured at the interval of 10 min, 20 min, 30 min. 1. It is measured as percentage of blood flow increased at 30 min. 2. Area under curve (AUC).

Inflammation-induced by irritants in normal skin

Various chemicals used for inducing inflammation are capsaicin (highly pungent paprika applied in bandage), mustard oil (ointment), histamin (prick with the needle containing the drug)

Ultraviolet B rays-induced inflammation of human skin

Ultraviolet B rays are delivered on small area of the skin and degree of inflammation is assessed.

Harrison's Biglow method (ischemic pain)

Procedure: Healthy human volunteers are selected. They are asked to raise their arm above the shoulder levels followed by tying of sphygmomanometer cuff around the arm. The pressure in the cuff is raised 20–30 mmHg above the systolic blood pressure. Then the participants are subjected to exercise, i.e. squeezing of cotton ball (to induce the ischaemic pain). Time required to feel the pain before and after taking the drug.

EVALUATION OF ANTIPEPTIC ULCER DRUGS

Introduction

Peptic ulcer results due to an imbalance between the aggressive and the defensive factors. Aggressive factors are gastric acid, pepsin, bile and *H. pylori*. Defensive factors are gastric mucus and bicarbonate secretion, prostaglandins, nitric oxide, innate resistance of the mucosal cells. Peptic ulcer occurs in that part of the gastrointestinal tract which is exposed to gastric acid, i.e. the stomach and duodenum. A variety of psychosomatic, humoral and vascular derangements have been implicated and the importance of *Helicobacter pylori* infection as a contributor to ulcer formation and recurrence has been recognized.

Various new drugs are coming for the treatment of peptic ulcer, hence it is important to learn the various methods use for evaluation of peptic ulcer.

In vivo Methods

1. **Antisecretory method:**
   - Whole stomach preparation in rat (Ghosh and Schild method)
   - Isolated whole stomach preparation in rat
2. **Gastric antiulcer activity**
   - Pylorus ligation in rat/Shay et.al
   - *Stress ulcer*—restrain induced, cold water immersion + restraint, and swimming
   - Histamine-induced gastric ulcer in guinea pig
   - Ethyl alcohol-induced gastric ulcer
   - Acetic acid-induced gastric ulcer
3. **Duodenal ulcer**
   - Cysteamine induced
   - Damaprit induced
   - Mepirizole induced
4. **Cytoprotective**

Duodenal Ulcer

1. **Cysteamine induced:** This method is used widely in evaluation of H2 blockers, anticholinergics, etc. Cysteamine reduces mucus production and increases gastric acid production.This method is described by Selye and Szabo.

   Procedure: Experimental animals are female Sprague-Dawley rats. Animals are divided in test and control groups. Cysteamine can be administered by oral/subcutaneous route. Animals are sacrified after 24 hours and 48 hours in oral and subcutaneous route respectively. Ulcerations will be seen on anterior wall of duodenum. Comparison is done in test and control group.

2. **Damaprit-induced duodenal ulcer:** It is a H2 receptor antagonist used for evaluation of H2 blockers. Multiple subcutaneous injections of damaprit (every hour for 6 hours) can cause gastric and duodenal ulcerations. Female Sprague-Dawley rats are used for the experiments. Animals are kept fasting for 24 hours. In test group drug under evaluation is administered 30 minutes before the administration of damaprit. Animal is sacrified after 6 hours. Comparison is done between test and control groups.

3. **Mepirizole-induced duodenal ulceration:** Mepirizole is a NSAID. This method is also used for study of pathogenesis of duodenal ulcers.

   Mepirizole is administered by oral route. In control group drug under evaluation is started 24 hours after mepirizole. Animal is sacrified on 11th day.

Gastric Antiulcer Activity

Gastric Ulcer by Stress Induction

Stress plays an important role in the pathogenesis of gastric ulcer. Ease of gastric acid production made it popular over the pylorus ligation.

1. **Restraint-induced ulcers:** In this method albino rats are used as experimental animal. Animal is kept fasting for 36 hours. Animal is subjected to restraint by moulding in specialised steel window screen and to prevent movement

the limbs are tied in the pairs. The restraint period is for 24 hours. Stomach is dissected out after scarificing the animal. Ulcer index and severity is calculated and compared in both groups.

2. **Stress-induced ulcer:** Various methods which can be used to induce stress ulcer are cold water immersion, NSAID and restraint. Parameters for observation in the following methods are ulcer severity and ulcer index.

Ulcer severity is graded as 0 = no ulcer, 1 = superficial, 2= deep, 3 = perforation

Ulcer index is summation of percentage of animals with ulcer, number of ulcers and severity of ulcers.

a. *Stress induction by restraint and cold water immersion:* Cold water immersion with additional restraint will accelerate the process of ulceration and reduce the period of immobilisation. Restraint period is for 16 hours and immersed in cold water at 22°C for 1 hour. Animal is scarificed after 24 hours.

b. *Stress-induced by swimming:* Albino rats are used as experimental animals. Animals are kept fasting for 24 hours later on subjected for swimming for 5 hours at 23°C in tube. The stomach is dissected out after scarificing the animal.

c. *Stress and NSAID:* Stress is induced by immersion 23°C for 7 hours. NSAID (aspirin, indomethacin, diclofenac) is given intraperitoneally, which is followed by immersion. Animals are then sacrificed and ulcer index calculated.

Chemical Induced Gastric Ulcers

a. **Histamine induced:** Widely used model. Experimental animal guinea pig fasted 36 hours. Injection histamine 50 mg IV. Injection promethazine intraperitoneally 5 mg given 50 min before and after histamine. 4 hours after histamine injection animal is sacrificed.

b. **Ethanol induced:** In this method absolute ethyl alcohol is used for ulcer induction. Experimental animals are wistar rats. Animals are kept fasting for 18 hours but water is given *ad libitum*. In test group drug under evaluation is given and 30 minutes later absolute alcohol 1 ml is given orally. After 1 hour animal is scarified and stomach is dissected out and studied for ulceration. Comparison between two groups gives the protection offered by drug.

c. **Acetic acid induced:** Experimental animal albino rats 0.05 ml acetic acid (1–30%) is given in sub-mucosal layer of stomach. Penetrating peptic ulcers with adhesions to the surrounding organs like liver.

d. **Reserpine:** Experimental animal Sprague-Dawley rats. Reserpine stimulated release of histamine from mast cells. It is administered by intraperitoneal route at a dose of 5 mg/kg.

e. **Cysteamine induced:** Inhibition mucus production, increased gastrin, prolongation of gastric emptying time. 10 % cysteamine given as 20 mg/100 gm by subcutaneous route twice at a gap of 4 hours.

f. Other chemical like dimaprit (H2 receptor agonist) and meperizole (NSAID) are also used.

Anti-secretory Method

Whole Stomach Preparation in Rat (Ghosh and Schild Method)

Ghosh and Schild perfused rat stomach preparation

Experimental animal: Rat (Sprague-Dawley/Wistar)

Procedure: The rats are fasted overnight *ad libitum* for 18 hours. Animals are anaesthetized with urethane solution. A heating pad is used to maintain the body temperature. Trachea is exposed and cannulated for artificial respiration, external jugular vein is cannulated. Open the abdomen with a midline incision and expose the pyloric end of the stomach and cannulate it. The stomach is washed with sodium hydroxide and the perfusate flows through a microflow glass electrode which is in turn connected to a pH meter and to an ink recorder. Changes in the acid secretion are noted as in the pH meter. This method can be applied for secretogogues like pentagastrin, histamine and carbochol.

Pylorus Ligation in Rat (Shay et al)

If stomach mucosa comes in contact with gastric acid for long period result in ulceration of mucosa. This can be done by ligation of pylorus part of stomach.

Preparation: Animal should be fasted for 48 hours. Water can be given *ad libitum*. Animal should be housed in individually.

EVALUATION OF ANTI-INFLAMMATORY

Introduction

It the protective response of the body for harmful stimuli. It involves the complex pathways with various components like cells, cytokines and antibodies.

Three phases of inflammation are:
- Phase 1 (acute phase): Increase vascular permeability
- Phase 2 (subacute): Leucocyte infiltration
- Phase 3 (chronic): Cellular proliferation

Drugs used are:
1. NSAIDs (nonsteroidal anti-inflammatory drugs)
2. Steroids

Experimental models are divided as
1. Animal models for acute and sub-acute inflammation
2. Animal models for chronic inflammation

Acute and Sub-acute Inflammation

1. Carrageenan-induced rat paw oedema
2. Carrageenan-induced pluresy
3. Croton oil-induced ear oedema
4. Oxozolone-induced oedema in guinea pig
5. Ultraviolet rays-induced erythema in guinea pig
6. Air pouch in rat

Chronic Inflammation

1. Cotton pellete granuloma
2. Glass rod granuloma
3. Adjuvant arthritis
4. Sponge implantation

Experimental Models for Acute Inflammation

Rat Paw Edema Test

Experimental animal: Sprague-Dawley rat/mice

  Chemicals: Carrageenan, bradykinin, 1% formalin, kaolin, egg albumin

  Equipment: Plethysmograph filled with mercury

  Procedure: Injection of carragenin is injected in the hindpaw. Anti-inflammatory drug is given by oral route half an hour prior to the injection of irritant. In control animal only vehicle is given volume of paw is measured in control as well as test group by using plethysmograph. (volume indicates edema). Degree of inhibition of edema indicates anti-inflammatory activity.

Carrageenan-induced Pluresy

Experimental animals: Sprague-Dawley rat

Procedure

- **Injection of irritant in the pleural cavity:** Animal is anaesthetised and the irritant (2% of 1 ml carrageenan) is injected into the 7th–8th intercostal space.
- **Drug under evaluation is injected** intra-peritoneally 24 hours and 48 hours after the irritant and 1 hour before scarifying the animal.
- **Animal is sacrificed after 3 days.** Plural exudate is removed with the help of Hank's solution (maintain the integrity of cells)
  Parameter for observation: Volume of exudates

Croton Oil-induced Ear Oedema

It is obtained by crushing the seeds of *Croton tiglium*. Widely used for inducing ear oedema.

  Procedure: 75 µgm of croton oil is applied to the inner year. It is left for 6 hours. Then the animal is sacrificed. The circular part of ear pinna is punched out (6 mm diameter).

  Parameter for observation: Difference in the weight of tissue in control and test group.

Oxozolone-induced Oedema in Guinea Pig

Experimental animal: Guinea pig.

Chemical: 2% Oxozolone in acetone.

Procedure: Topically it is applied to the right ear. In the test group it is mixed with drug.

Parameter: After 8 days the animal is scarificed and the disc of 8 mm diameter is punched from both the ears. Weight is measured and compared.

Ultraviolet Rays-induced Erythema in Guinea Pig

Experimental animal: Guinea pig

Procedure: Animal is shaved 18 hours before the procedure followed by application of depilatory cream which is later rinsed off. The animals are pre-treated with the test drug half an hour before UV exposure from a UV lamp emitting radiation in the wavelength of 180–220 nm. Other body part is covered with leather coat with punch.

Results: Scoring system is applied (2 hours and 4 hours)

0 No erythema
1. Weak erythema
2. Strong erythema
3. Very erythema

Air Pouch-induced Acute Inflammation

Experimental animals: Sprague-Dawely rat/mice

Procedure: Subcutaneous dorsal pouches are created in anaesthetised mice by injecting 5 ml of air. After 3 days the pouches are re-injected with the carrageenan in sterile saline. 24 hours after injection animals are sacrificed.

Test drug is administered 30 minutes before 8 hours and 20 hours after carrageenan by oral route. Pouches are washed and exudates are studied for anti-inflammatory action.

EVALUATION OF ANTI-INFLAMMATORY DRUGS FOR CHRONIC INFLAMMATION

1. Cotton pellet granuloma   2. Adjuvant arthritis

Cotton Pellet Granuloma

Experimental animal: Rat

Procedure: Sterile weighed cotton is implanted subcutaneously in the plantar aspect of foot in the rat. After seven days, the granuloma (it is a foreign body reaction to cotton pellet) is formed. During this period of seven days rats are administered vehicle in control group and drug under evaluation is administered in test group. On the 8th day granuloma is dissected out under anaesthesia. Weight of the granuloma is estimated in both the groups (initial weight is subtracted from total weight at 8th day). Difference in weight of granuloma in control group and treated group gives estimate of anti-inflammatory activity.

Adjuvant Arthritis

Experimental animal: Rat

Procedure: Arthritis is induced by subcutaneous injection of Freund's complete adjuvant (mycobacteria suspended in oil). Followed by sub-plantar injection of Freund's complete adjuvant in the volume of 50–100 μl. There will be swelling of the paw on same side within 24 hours and systemic disease will appear after 10–12 days. This is in the form of swelling on quantra-lateral side.

EVALUATION OF ANTICANCER DRUGS

Cancer is a disease in which abnormal cells divide uncontrollably and destroy the body tissues. The goal of screening models in cancer is to identify compounds that kill cancer cells and have the ability to discriminate the proliferating and non-proliferating cells. Different properties of cells are utilized to study anticancer properties.

IN VITRO METHODS

1. **MTT (Micro-culture tetrazolium test) assay:** It is the most commonly used assay for screening anti-cancer drugs.

    Principle: It is a colorimetric assay to identify living cells from nonviable or dead cells. The living cells convert a colourless substrate into a coloured product. A multi-well plate scanning spectrophotometer is used to quickly measure a large number of samples in a precise and accurate manner. The colour reaction which is used as a measure of viable cells in this assay is:

- Tetrazolium salt mitochondrial dehydrogenase formazan (blue)
- Intensity of blue coloured formazan is directly proportional to the number of viable cells. The advantage of this assay is that multiple samples can be analysed at one time and various drug concentrations can be analysed to obtain a DRC and IC50 (concentration of drug required to inhibit 50% of the cell growth) of each drug. It is simple, cheap, less time consuming used for both adherent and suspension cell lines.

2. **Sulforodamine B assay:** It measures protein content in culture medium. Proteins are stained by SRB which is a bright pink anionic dye. This assay is used to measure the cellular protein content of both adherent and suspension cultures.

3. **3H-thymidine uptake test:** The tumour cell suspensions are exposed to the drug for 5 days continuosly followed by which 3H-thymidine is added. The replicating cells incorporate 3H-thymidine and the nonreplicating cells will not be counted. It is a rapid and low maintenance assay.

4. **Fluorescence:** Fluorescent dyes are used *in vitro*. The cells are exposed to fluorescent labelled precursors after drug exposure. Replicating cells incorporate labelled precursor into their DNA and the fluorescence obtained is measured in flow cytometry.

5. **Clonogenic assays:** This assay measures loss of tumour cell reproductive viability. It is a direct method of measuring cytotoxic activity of the drug.

6. **Cell counting assay:** The cells are cultured in the presence of the drug for 2–5 culture doubling time followed by which the number of cells are counted using a hemocytometer or a cell counter. This assay is simple and can be used both for adherent and suspension cells.

In vivo Models

They are more useful than *in vitro* methods for screening anticancer drugs because they detect host mediated activity and estimate therapeutic ratio. The two most commonly employed methods are chemical induced and cell line induced tumour models.

DMBA-induced Mouse Skin Papillomas

Experimental animal: Mouse

The dorsal surface of the mice is shaven. Skin papillomas are induced by using DMBA and 12-O-tetradecanoyl-phorbol-13-acetate (TPA) which are applied as a single dose on the shaven back followed by a higher dose twice weekly. They are used as an inducer and a promoter respectively. Repeated topical application of DMBA alone also induces carcinogenesis.

N-methyl, N-nitrosourea (MNU)-induced Rat Mammary Gland Carcinogenesis

Experimental animal: Rat

Tumours are induced in rats by giving single IV injections of MNU. Tumours produced by MNU are adenocarcinomas. They are good models for breast cancer. Drug efficacy is measured as the percent reduction in the adenoma incidence, percent increase in adenocarcinoma latency compared to carcinogen control.

MNU-induced Tracheal Squamous Cell Carcinoma in Hamster

Experimental animal: Syrian golden hamster

A defined area of the trachea of syrian male hamster is exposed to 5% solution of MNU in normal saline with the help of specially designed catheters. The drug is administered once a week for 15 weeks followed by which tumours are produced in 40–50% of the animals within a period of 6–7 months. Efficacy of the test drug is measured as percentage reduction of tumour incidence compared with the carcinogenic control.

Other *in vivo* Models

- N, N-Diethylnitrosamine (DEN)-induced lung adeno-carcinoma in hamster
- DMBA-induced oral cancer in hamsters
- Hepatocellular cancer
- Pancreatic cancer models

CELL LINE TUMOUR PIECES IMPLANTATION

1. Hollow fiber technique
2. Use of xenografts

3. Nude mice models
4. Newborn Rat Model
5. Transgenic mouse model

Hollow Fiber Techniques

Experimental animal: Mouse

Cells from the human tumours are inserted under the skin and in the body cavity of the mouse with the help of small hollow fibers measuring a millimetre in diameter. Drugs are administered in two dosages and tested for 12 target tumours in different hollow tubes. Compounds which prevent the growth of the cells are used for the next level of testing. This test is done for 3–4 days.

Use of Xenografts

Experimental animal: Mouse

The skin of the mice is injected with human tumours directly. The drugs which proved to retard growth of cells in the hollow tubes are used. The drugs which retard the growth of specific tumour cells with minimal toxicity are used for the next level of testing.

Nude Mice Models

Experimental animal: Mice

Nude mice are devoid of thymus gland. They also lack helper T cells and tumour suppressor cells. They do not reject transplanted material. They are maintained in strict sterile conditions in warm environment. They are very expensive models. They can also be used for testing tumours like melanomas and carcinoma of colon.

Newborn Rat Model

Experimental animal: Rat pups

The cost effectiveness and low maintenance feature makes this a more feasible model. They are used for transplantation of tumours alternate to the nude mice models. Rat pups are used to study neural tumours. The animals are checked for palpable tumours twice weekly.

Transgenic Mouse Model

Experimental animal: Mouse

A genetically engineered metamouse is used. The tumour pieces from the patients are transplanted into the animal. Tumour of the liver, pancreas, neck and bladder develop well in a metamouse. It also serves as a surrogate marker in cancer patients.

The conventional methods of drug screening is being continuously refined with newer methods which helps in acceleration of the drug development process. Newer methods are being searched for to screen potential anticancer drugs.

ANTI-FERTILITY SCREENING

Anti-fertility agents are the agents which prevent the fertility by interfering with various normal reproductive mechanisms, in both males and females.

Methods for Females

1. Inhibition of ovulation
2. Prevention of fertilization
3. Interference with transport of ova from oviduct to endometrium of the uterus
4. Interference with the implantation of the fertilized ovum
5. Distraction of early implanted embryo

A. Antiovulatory Activity

* HCG-induced ovulation in rats
* Cupric acetate-induced ovulation in rabbits

B. Estrogenic Activity

* Vaginal opening
* Assay for water intake
* Vaginal cornification
* Chick oviduct method

In vitro Methods

* Estrogenic receptor binding assay
* Dextran coated charcoal (DCC)

C. Progestational Activity

In vivo Methods

- Pregnancy maintenance test
- Clauberg-McPhail test
- Prevention of abortion in oxytocin treated pregnant rabbits

D. Antiprogestational Activity

1. Anti-progestational activity in immature rabbits (Mac Ginty)
2. Anti-implantation activity
3. Abortifacient activity

Screening of Antifertility Agents in Males

1. **Sperm count and function**
   - *In vivo:* Cohabitation test, subsidiary test
   - *In vitro:* Spermicidal activity, immobilization assay, nonspecific aggregation and estimation, sperm revival test, plasma membrane integrity, acrosomal status.
2. **Androgenic and antiandrogenic activity:** Chicken comb method, weight of ventral prostate, seminal vesicles and levatorani muscle.

A. Antiovulatory Activity

1. HCG-induced ovulation in rats: Immature female albino rats do not ovulate spontaneously and hence priming with human chorionic gonadotropin (HCG) induces follicular maturation leading to spontaneous ovulation after 2 days. Injection of anti-ovulatory drugs, prior to the induction procedure will prevent ovulation.
2. Cupric acetate induced ovulation in rabbits: Rabbits being reflex ovulators; ovulate within a few hours after mating or even in the presence of males or administration of chemical like cupric acid. Here cupric acetate is used as an ovulation inducing agent. Injection of antiovulatory drugs, 24 hours before the induction procedure prevents ovulation.

B. Estrogenic Activity

Estrogen is used as contraception. Excess exogenous estrogen inhibits FSH and LH, thus preventing ovulation.

In vivo Methods

1. *Vaginal opening*
   Principle: Vaginal opening occurs in immature female albino mice and rats by treating them with estrogenic compounds. Complete vaginal opening is observed as a sign of estrogenic activity.

2. *Assay for water intake*
   Principle: Uterus responds to estrogen by increase uptake and retention of water. An increase in the water uptake is observed at six hours after administration of the drug.

   Immature rat or mice is used. The animals are randomly grouped. Test group is given oestrogen and control group is given 0.1 ml of cotton seed oil. The animals are sacrificed after 5 hours and the uterus is excised and kept damp on a dry filter paper and later weighed in a balance. They are dried and reweighed and the percentage increase in water over the control is calculated.

3. *Vaginal cornification:* Rats and mice exhibit a cyclical ovulation along with changes in the secretion of hormones leading to changes in vaginal epithelium. Drugs with estrogenic activity change the animals into estrus stage. The estrus cycle of a rat is completed in four to five days which include proestrus, estrus, metestrus and diestrus.

4. *Chick oviduct method:* The weight of the oviduct of young chicken is increased by natural and synthetic estrogen.

In vitro Methods

1. Estrogenic receptor binding assay
2. Dextran coated charcoal (DCC)

C. Progestational Activity

In vivo Methods

1. *Pregnancy maintenance test:* Progesterone maintains pregnancy. Rats are ovariectomised on days 5/10/15 of pregnancy. Animals are treated with test and standard drugs. The pregnant rats are sacrificed and an average of living foetuses at the end of the experiment are compared with the test and control groups.

2. *Clauberg-McPhail test:* Rabbits are primed with estradiol followed by progestational compounds which lead to the

proliferation of endometrium and thus it is converted into secretary phase.

3. *Prevention of abortion in oxytocin treated pregnant rabbits:* Administration of oxytocin to pregnant rabbits on the 30th day of pregnancy causes abortion. Administration of progestational compounds prior to oxytocin prevents abortion.

   Pregnant rabbits are treated with IV oxytocin on the 30th day of pregnancy. Control group animals which are not treated with progesterone prior abort.

D. Antiprogestational Activity

The antiprogestational compounds inhibit physiological effects of progesterone.

Anti-progestational activity in immature rabbits (Mac Ginty)

Experimental animal: Immature rabbits

Principle: Immature rabbits primed with estrogen for 6 days. They are first exposed to local progesterone locally in the uterine segment in one uterine horn after giving anaesthesia. The opposite horn serves as control. The animal is sacrificed after 3 days and the uterus is evaluated histologically according to MacPhail's score. The scoring is done from 0 to 4 where zero denotes no proliferation and four denotes very pronounced proliferation and ramification of the uterine mucosa. Inhibition of proliferation of the uterine cavity is the index of antiprogestational activity.

E. Antiimplantation Activity

Experimental animal: Female albino rat

Principle: Mature male and female rats with established fertility are mated. Once mating is confirmed the female is caged singly and drug is administered orally daily. The animal is sacrificed after 10 days and the number of implants in both uterine horns and number of corpus lutea on each ovary is counted. The animals are allowed to complete the gestational period and the number of litter delivered are noted. The following parameters are evaluation: Preimplantation loss, post-implantation loss and antifertility activity was calculated.

F. Abortifacient Activity

Experimental animal: Female albino rabbits

Principle: The pregnant rabbit is exposed to test drug on 20th day of pregnancy by injecting it into the amniotic fluid or placenta or any any route. Effect of drug is seen by vaginal bleeding, changes in weight, abdominal palpation and post-mortem examination.

Screening of Antifertility Agents in Males

1. **Sperm count and function**
   - *In vivo*: Cohabitation test, subsidiary test
   - *In vitro*: Spermicidal activity, immobilization assay, non-specific aggregation and estimation, sperm revival test, plasma membrane integrity, acrosomal status.
2. **Androgenic and antiandrogenic activity:** Chicken comb method, weight of ventral prostate, seminal vescicles and levatorani muscle.

EVALUATION OF ANTIOBESITY DRUGS

Obesity is a medical condition in which excess fat accumulates in the body and have a negative effect on a person's health, leading to decreased life expectancy and increased health problems.

It is also defined as the body mass index (BMI) greater than 30 kg/m^2 and range of 25–30 kg/m is referred to as overweight. The global incidence of obesity is considered as one of the leading causes for morbidity and mortality in the current and the future generations. Various animal models are used for the study of factors causing obesity and for the discovery of various treatments for obesity.

The parameters studied in animal models are: Food intake, body weight, adipose tissue cell size and number, body composition, locomotor/physical activity, plasma lipids, insulin and glucose levels.

Classified as:

1. Diet-induced obesity
2. *Surgically induced and chemically induced:* Hypothalamic obesity

3. Virus-induced obesity
4. *Genetic models of obesity:* Monogenic and polygenic models

Diet-induced Obesity

Experimental animal: Adult female rats.

Procedure: House the animals weighing approximately 230 g in individual wire mess. Animals are grouped into test and control. Control group receives ordinary Purina cow; test group receives Purina cow, high fat diet, sweetened milk, cheese, peanut butter, etc. The parameters studied are body weight, food intake, locomotor activity and serum insulin in both the groups are compared.

Hypothalamic Obesity

Hypothalamus plays a very important role in regulating food intake by interaction of a lateral feeding centre and a medial satiety centre.

a. Surgically Induced

Experimental animal: Female Sprague-Dawley

Procedure: The animals are fed high fat diet for 5–9 days following which they are anaesthetized with pentobarbital sodium intraperitoneally. Hypothalamic lesions are produced by bilateral knife cuts. Sham operated rats serve as control. Parameters observed: Food intake, body weight and compared between test and control group.

b. Chemically Induced

Experimental animal: Mice, young albino rats

Chemicals used: Mono-sodium L glutamate, gold thioglucose implants, bipiperidyl mustard

The chemical is injected into the animal intraperitoneally or intra cerebrally and obesity is produced.

Virus-induced Obesity

Experimental animal: Mice, rats, chickens, nonhuman primates

Virus used: Canine distemper virus, borna disease virus, avian adenovirus SMAM-I

Animals are infected with the virus which leads to development of obesity after 8–10 days of infection. The exact mechanism of virus-induced obesity is not clear.

Genetic Models of Obesity

Monogenic models: They are the naturally arising mutations causing obesity.

Animal	Description
Yellow obese mouse	Mutation in chromosome 2 They exhibit moderate obesity and diabetes
Obese mouse	Mutation in chromosome 6 Characterized by obesity, hyperglycemia and insulin resistance
Diabetic mouse	Mutation in chromosome 4 They exhibit marked obesity, hyperglycemia and insulin resistance
Fat mouse	Model of late onset obesity Fat mutation on chromosome 8 They exhibit hyperinsulinemia, obesity, infertility
Tubby mouse	Tub mutation They exhibit slow onset obesity, sensorineural hearing loss and retinal degeneration
Fatty rat	• Most widely used rat model • It is a cross between Sherman and Merck stock M rats
Obese SHR rat	• It is developed by mating a spontaneously hypertensive female rat with a normotensive Sprague-Dawley male rat

Polygenic models: They resemble human obesity phenotypes than single gene models. They have multiple genetic loci within individual strains that modify obesity, plasma cholesterol levels and they can also develop obesity on a high fat diet.

Models	Description
Otsuka-Long-Evans-Tokushima fatty rats	• Maintained at the Tokushima Research Institute, Japan • Characterized by mild obesity, hyperglycemia, polyuria and polydipsia
Japanese KK mouse	• They exhibit hyperinsulinemia, hyperphagia and moderate hyperglycemia
NZO mouse (New Zealand obese)	• They develop obesity, mild hyperglycemia and insulin resistance

Transgenic or knockout animal models:
1. Knockout of β_3 adrenergic receptor gene
2. Knockout of uncoupling protein in brown adipose tissue
3. Knockout mice lacking steroidgenic factor

EVALUATION OF DRUGS FOR BRONCHIAL ASTHMA

Asthma is a chronic, heterogeneous inflammatory disorder of the airways characterized by reversible airway obstruction, inflammation and bronchial hyper-responsiveness. Among several respiratory diseases, bronchial asthma is the most common disabling syndrome.

Various models and screening method used for evaluation of bronchial asthma drugs are as follows.

In vitro **methods**
1. Isolated tracheal chain-spasmolytic activity in guinea pig
2. Isolated lung strips
3. Isolated lung perfusion in closed system
4. Inhibition of histamine release from mast cells

In vivo **methods**
1. Broncho-spasmolytic activity in anaesthetized guinea pig
2. Bronchial hyper reactivity
   a. Histamine-induced spasm in guinea pig
   b. Histamine-induced spasm in anaesthetized guinea pig
3. Systemic anaphylaxis in rat
4. Anti-anaphylaxis in guinea pig
5. Passive cutaneous anaphylaxis in rat
6. Delayed type of hypersensitivity

In vitro Method

1. **Isolated tracheal chain:** Spasmolytic activity in guinea pig
   Experimental animal: Guinea pig
   Procedure: Guinea pig is sacrificed by using ether anaesthesia. The entire trachea is dissected out. Individual tracheal rings are isolated. 12–15 rings are tied together with silk thread. Tracheal rings are mounted in the organ bath. **PSS is Krebs Hanslet solution,** temperature 37°C tension 0.5 gm with carbogen. Various spasmogens used

are **histamine, carbachol, LTC4**. Spasmogen is added and the contraction is noted. Relaxant effect of standard and test drug are recorded.

2. **Spasmolytic activity of guinea pig lung strips**

   Experimental animal: Guinea pig

   Procedure: Guinea pig is sacrificed by using ether anaesthesia. Lungs are isolated and cut into strips of 5 cm. Lung strips are mounted in the organ bath with PSS as Krebs Hanslet solution, temperature 37°C, preload 0.5–3 gm with carbogen. Various spasmogens used are histamine, carbachol, LTC4. Spasmogen is added and the contraction is noted. Relaxant effect of standard and test drug are recorded.

3. **Isolated lung perfusion in closed system**

   Experimental animal: Guinea pig

   Principle: Change in the air volume of a living animal in a closed system consisting of respiratory pump, trachea and bronchi are measured. A decrease in the volume of inspired air and increase in residual volume is induced by bronchoconstriction.

   Procedure: Guinea pigs are anaesthetized with urathrane intraperitonially. Animals are put on artificial respiration by cannulating the trachea and connecting to respiratory pump. Artificial respiration is given with 60 strokes/min. Excess air not taken by lungs is measured and recorded in a polygraph. Drugs are administered through internal jugular vein. Each animal is placed in a plastic container with 15 litre volume. Bronchospasm is induced by 0.5 solution of histamine in aerosol form for 5 minutes.

In vivo **Methods**

1. **Bronchospasmolytic activity in anaesthetized guinea pig**

   Experimental animal: guinea pig

   Procedure: Anaesthetized with uratrane 1.25 gm/kg ip Animals are put on artificial respiration by cannulating the trachea and connecting to respiratory pump. Artificial respiration is given with 60 strokes/min. Excess air not taken by lungs is measured and recorded in a polygraph. Drugs are administered through internal jugular vein and carotid artery is cannulated for blood pressure. Respiratory pump is connected to polygraph for measuring excess air not taken up by lungs. Each animal is placed in a plastic container with 15 litre volume. Various spasmogens used are histamine, ACh, bradykinin, LT. After administration of bronchospasmodic drug, the test compound is given by iv/sc route. Spasmogens are repeated at 15, 30, 60 mins and the effect is observed. Bronchospasm is induced by 0.5 solution of histamine in aerosol form for 5 minutes.

2. **Bronchial hyperreactivity**
   - Histamine-induced spasm in guinea pig
   - Experimental animal is guinea pig

   Procedure: Guinea pigs are pre-treated with test drug and controlled drugs. Animals pre-treated with test drug are exposed to the spasmogen like histamine in the form of aerosol. Parameter for observation is time required for hypoxia-induced convulsion. Test drug with bronchodilator property will offer protection from hypoxia.

   Other spasmogens: Bradykinin, PAF, serotonin and oval albumin—these are administered by parenteral route. Vagal stimulation can be used to induce bronchospasm.

3. **Micro-shock in Rabbit**

   Experimental animal: Rabbit

   Procedure: Rabbits are placed in a close chamber with open side down on a smooth rubber surface. It is connected to a nebulizer for delivery of 0.2% histamine aerosol. Dose of the histamine aerosol is increased gradually. In minor doses it shows a symptom like shock called micro-shock. This includes increase respiratory rate, then it becomes laborious and further exposure cause convulsions, urination, cyanosis and death. Test drug is administered intraperitoneally 30 minutes before the procedure. Preconvulsion time is recorded. Percentage of protection given by the drug is calculated as $(1 - T1/T2) \times 100$.

   T1: Pre-convulsion time in control, T2: Pre-convulsion time after giving drug.

ANTIDIABETIC SCREENING

Diabetes mellitus is a metabolic disorder characterized by abnormal carbohydrate, protein, fat metabolism caused by the complete or relative insufficiency of insulin secretion and/or insulin action.

Experimental induction of diabetes mellitus in animals is done for better understanding of the various aspects of its pathogenesis and ultimately finding new therapies and cure.

Animal models are classified as:

1. **Chemical induced**
   - Streptozocin induced
   - Alloxan induced
   - Gold thioglucose (GTG) obese diabetic mouse model
   - Atypical antipsychotic induced
2. **Surgical induced**
   - Pancreactomised rat
3. **Genetic models**
   - Zuker diabetic fatty rat
   - GotoKakizaki (GK rat)
   - Db/db mice
   - Obese rhesus monkey
4. **Virus-induced models**
   - Coxsackie B4
   - Enchephalomyocarditis
   - Mengom–2T
   - Reo virus
   - LMCV
5. **Oral glucose loading animal model**
6. **Insulin antibodies induced diabetes**

Chemical Models

1. **Streptozocin-induced diabetes mellitus**
   Experimental animal: Rats, rabbit, primates

   Procedure: Streptozocin induces diabetes mellitus in the experimental animal by causing degeneration of beta cells of pancreas. It can be given single/multi dose injections. It induces diabetes in 2–4 days. Other animals used in this experimental model are rabbit, primates.

2. **Alloxan-induced diabetes mellitus**
   Experimental animal: Rat

   Procedure: Alloxan is widely used to induce type 2 diabetes in animals. Alloxan causes triphasic response in

animals. Stage I—early hyperglycemia of short duration about 1–4 hr due to a sudden short lasting decrease or cessation of insulin release and direct glycogenolytic effects on the liver. Stage II—hyperglycemia phase lasting up to 48 hours and often resulting in convulsion and death. Stage III—chronic diabetic phase consequence of insulin lack histologically, only a few ß cells if any are detectable in animals with fully developed alloxan diabetes.

3. **Goldthioglucose (GTG) obese diabetic mouse model**
   Experimental animal: Mice

   Procedure: Type 2 diabetes with obesity can be induced in mice by intraperitonial injection of goldthioglucose. The animal gradually develops obesity, hyperinsulinaemia, hyperglycemia, insulin resistance over a period of 16–20 weeks after GTG injection. The GTG causes venteromedical hypothalamic nucleus necrotic lesions, which subsequently are responsible for the development of overeating and obesity.

4. **Atypical antipsychotic-induced diabetic model**
   Experimental animal: Rat

   *Proceudure:*Atypical antipsychotic agents are associated with the emergence of severe metabolic adverse effect like glucose deregulation, insulin resistance, hyperlipidemia, weight gain and hypertension.

   Atypical antipsychotics which can be used for the study are clozapine, olanzapine, risperidone, ziprasidone or haloperidol. Techniques used in this experiments are hyperinsulinemic-euglycemic and hyperglycemic clamp procedures. Clozapine and olanzapine had a rapid and potent effect on insulin sensitivity by increasing hepatic glucose production and decreased peripheral glucose utilization. Neither ziprasidone nor haloperidol had a significant impact on insulin sensitivity.

5. **Surgically-induced diabetes mellitus**
   • **Pancreatectomy in dogs**
     Experimental animal: Beagle dog

     Procedure: Male Beagle dogs are anaesthetized with an intravenous injection of 50 mg/kg pentobarbital sodium and placed on its back. Abdomen is opened by midline incision. A self-retaining retractor is applied. By passing the right hand along the stomach to the pylorus, the duodenum with the head of the pancreas is brought into the operating field. All the glandular tissue being attached very firmly has to be carefully removed in order to leave no residual pancreatic tissue behind. The pancreatic duct is cleaned, doubly ligated and cut between the ligatures. The dissection proceeds until one encounters a small lobe containing the main pancreatic duct. The glandular tissue adheres here firmly to the duodenum.

- **Non-obese partial pancreatectomised diabetic animals**: This model is suitable for studying the effects of locally produced insulin on pancreatic exocrine function in metabolically normal animals.
- **Duodenal-jejunal bypass non-obese T-2 DM**: This model has shown to reverse T-2 DM in GK rats.

6. **Insulin antibody-induced diabetes mellitus**

   Experimental animal: Guinea pig

   Procedure: Insulin antibodies are produced by injection of bovine insulin along with the CFA to a guinea pig. Guinea pig antiserum is injected by intravenous route to the guinea pig in the dose of 0.25 ml to 1 ml. Large doses produce ketonemia, ketonuria, glycosuria and acidosis.

7. **Oral glucose loading animal model**

   Experimental animal: Rat/mice

   Procedure: Blood glucose level is transiently increased in the animal with no damage to the pancreas when diabetes mellitus is induced physiologically. It is also called oral glucose tolerance test which has been widely used for the diagnosis of impaired glucose tolerance, diabetes mellitus and gestational diabetes.

Genetic Models

Zukker diabetic fatty rat: Inbreeding of a substrain of fa/fa (leptin receptor deficient) rats that exhibit hyperglycemia. These animals develop obesity, insulin resistance and overt NIDDM between 7 and 10 weeks of age.

Goto-Kakizaki rat: It is a genetic model of type 2 DM characterized by nonobesity, moderate but stable fasting hyperglycemia, hypoinsulinaemia, normolipidemia, impaired glucose tolerance appearing at 2 weeks of age along with early onset of diabetic complications.

Obese rhesus monkeys: An excellent nonrhodent model develops obesity, hyperinsulinemia and insulin resistance.

Virus induced diabetic model: Various human viruses used for inducing diabetes include RNA picorna virus, coxsakie B4, encephalomylocarditis, reovirus.

TABLE 9.1: Advantages and disadvantages of different categories of diabetic models

Model	Advantage	Disadvantage
Chemical	Selectively damage beta cells (no alpha and delta cells lost)	Direct damage to beta cells, hence hyperglycemia is induced by insulin deficiency
	Residual insiulin secretrion is intact, mortality is less	No effect on insulin resistance can be tested
		Results are variable
	Comparatively cheaper, easier to develop and maintain	Beta cell damage is unstable
		Can be regenerated, hence unsuitable for long-term experiment
Surgical	No cytotoxic effect on other body part	Cumbersome and difficult
		Postoperative problems
		High mortality
		Loss of alpha and delta cells
Genetic	All genetic factors are considered	Sophisticated and costly

BIBLIOGRAPHY

1. NS Parmar, Shiv Prakash, Screening Methods in Pharmacology, New Delhi, Narosa Publishing House, Laboratory animal, 37.
2. SK Gupta, Drug Screening Methods (Preclinical evaluation of new drugs), New Delhi, Jaypee Brothers, Second edition 2009.
3. Vogel HG et al, Drug discovery and evaluation: Methods in clinical Pharmacology, Germany, Springer Publication House.

CPCSEA Guidelines

INTRODUCTION

- Good laboratory practices (GLP) for animal facilities assures quality maintenance and safety of animals used in laboratory studies while conducting biomedical and behavioural research and testing of products.

Goals of Committee for the Purpose of Control and Supervision on Experiments on Animals (CPCSEA)

- Provide humane care of animals used in biomedical, behavioural research and testing of products.
- Provide specifications that will enhance animal welfare.

Veterinary Care

- Adequate veterinary care should be provided by the veterinarian.
- Daily observations of the animals for their behaviour, health and well being.
- Help in reviewing protocols and proposals, animal husbandry and animal welfare; monitoring occupational health hazards containment, and zoonosis control programs.

Animal Procurement

- Animals are procured and transported as per committee for the purpose of control and supervision on experiments on animals (CPCSEA) guidelines.

- A health surveillance program to check for the quality of animals is conducted.

Quarantine, Stabilizing and Separation

- Separation of newly procured animals to minimize the introduction of pathogens into the already established colony and
- Minimum duration of quarantine
  Small animals: 1 week
  Large animals: 6 weeks
- *Physical separation of animals:* To prevent interspecies transmission of diseases.

Surveillance, Diagnosis, Treatment and Control of Disease

- Animals should be observed for signs of illness, injury, or abnormal behaviour.
- *Unexpected deaths and signs of illness, distress, or other deviations from normal health condition in animals:* Should be reported promptly and appropriate veterinary medical care should be provided.
- Animals showing signs of a contagious disease should be isolated from healthy animals in the colony.

Animal Care and Technical Personnel

- Institutions must employ people trained in laboratory animal science, provide them training to ensure effective implementation of the program.

Personal Hygiene

- Animal care staff must maintain a high standard of personal cleanliness.
- Facilities for shower, change of uniforms, footwear, gloves, masks, head covers, coats, coveralls and shoe covers should be available.
- No permission to eat, drink, smoke or apply cosmetics in animal rooms.

Animal Experimentation involving Hazardous Agents

- Institutional biosafety committee and the institutional animal ethics committee examines the proposal and the procedures to be conducted.

Multiple Surgical Procedures on Single Animal

• Multiple procedures are not practised unless it is specified in the protocol and approved by the IAEC.

Duration of Experiments

• Not more than 3 years.

Physical Restraint

• Done for experimentations, collection of samples, experimental manipulations.
• Prolonged restraint should be avoided.
• Veterinary care should be provided if lesions or illness associated with restraint are observed.

Physical Plant

• A well-planned, properly maintained facility is an important element in good animal care.

Physical Relationship of Animal Facilities to Laboratories

• Isolated from human habitation.
• The animals housing area should be placed near the laboratory.

Functional Areas

• Ensure separation of species or isolation of individual projects when necessary.
• Receive, quarantine, and isolate animals.
• Availability of specialized laboratories.

Physical Facilities

Facilities	Description
Building materials	• Durable, moisture-proof, fire-resistant, seamless materials are most desirable for interior surfaces including vermin and pest resistance
Corridor	• Should be wide enough and kept clean
Utilities	• Water lines, drain pipes and electrical connections should preferably be accessible through service panels or shafts in corridors outside the animal rooms.
Animal room doors	• Rust, dust and vermin free • Rodent barriers may be provided

Contd.

Facilities	Description
Exterior windows	• *Small animal facilities*: Not recommended • *Primates*: Recommended
Floor	• Maintained with wet vaccuming or mopping with disinfectants • Drainage must be adequate to allow rapid removal of water and drying of surfaces
Walls and ceilings	• Crack free
Storage area	• Separate storage areas should be designed for feed, bedding, cages and materials not in use.
Facilities for sanitizing equipment and supplies	• An area for sanitizing cages and ancillary equipment is essential with adequate water supply
Experimental area	• Experimental procedures for small animals should be conducted in a separate room away from the animal house. • *Large animals*: Separate surgical room, with aseptic precautions
Environment a. Temperature and humidity control	• Air conditioning should be made available • Temperature and humidity control helps prevent variations due to changing climatic conditions
b. Ventilation	• Adequate ventilation should be provided
c. Power and lighting	• Appropriate lighting, illumination and a sufficient number of power outlets should be provided • Emergency power should be available in case of power failure
d. Noise control	• Noise tree premises should be maintained • Concrete walls are efficient in reducing the efficiency of sound transmission
Animal husbandry a. Caging or housing system	• Caging and housing system should be designed carefully to facilitate animal well-being, meet research requirements, and minimize experimental variables • A comfortable environment, escape proof enclosure that confines animal safety, adequate ventilation should be maintained
Sheltered or outdoor housing	• Adequate protection from extremes in temperature or other harsh weather conditions and adequate protective. • Ground-level surfaces of outdoor housing facilities can be covered with absorbent bedding, sand, gravel so that it can be removed or replaced when needed to ensure adequate sanitation.

Activity

- Provisions for animals to express their locomotor patterns should be made available. For example, ropes, bars.
- Cages should be provided for post-surgical care.
- Pens, runs, or other out-of-cage space should be provided to increase the opportunity for exercise.

Food

- Animals should be fed palatable, non-contaminated, and nutritionally adequate food daily.
- Animal food store should be kept clean and enclosed to prevent entry of insects or other animals.
- Exposure to extremes in relative humidity, unsanitary conditions, light, oxygen, and insects hasten the deterioration of food.

Bedding

- Should be absorbent and toxin free.
- Bedding should be replaced as and when required to keep the animals clean and dry.
- Nesting materials for newly delivered pups wherever can be provided (e.g. paper, tissue paper and cotton).

Water

- Continuous access to fresh, potable, uncontaminated drinking waters should be provided.
- Microbial contamination of water should be prevented and periodic monitoring is done to check for contamination.

Sanitation and Cleanliness

- Maintaining sanitation is an essential component of the animal house.
- Detergents and disinfectants are used to clean the premises to keep the animal house away from dirt, dust, debris.
- Cages should be sanitized before placing the animals in them.
- Water bottles, sipper tubes, stoppers, and other watering equipment should be washed and then sanitized by rinsing with water or hyperchlorite.
- Adequate pest control is provided to prevent infestations by pests.

Waste Disposal

- Should be removed regularly, and should be disposed off in a safe and sanitary method in disposable and leakproof liners.

Emergency, Weekend and Holiday Care

- Animals should be taken care of even during emergency and holidays.

Record Keeping

- Records of the following data should be maintained: Animal house plans, animal house staff record—both technical and non-technical, health record of staff/animals, all standard operating procedures (SOPs) relevant to the animals.
- Breeding, stock, purchase and sales records, minutes of Institute Animals Ethics Committee Meetings, records of experiments conducted with the number of animals used (copy of Form D) and death record clinical record of sick animals.

Personnel and Training

- In-house training for staff at all levels must be provided.
- Regular medical check up for the staff to check for any zoonotic diseases.

Transport of Laboratory Animals

- Transport of animals must be done with utmost care.
- Food and water must be made available to the animals.

Anaesthesia

The animal is prepared for anaesthesia by overnight fasting and using pre-anaesthetics

- The animal should remain under veterinary care till it completely recovers from anaesthesia and postoperative stress.

Euthanasia

- Euthanasia is resorted to events where an animal is required to be sacrificed on termination of an experiment or otherwise for ethical reasons.
- The method should be humane.

• Death, without causing anxiety, pain or distress with minimum time lag phase, with minimum physiological and psychological disturbances.

Transgenic Animals

• A transgenic animal is one that carries a foreign gene that has been deliberately inserted into its genome.
• It can either developed in the laboratory or produced for R and D purpose from registered scientific/academic institutions or commercial firms, and generally from abroad with approval from appropriate authorities.
• Special care has to be taken with transgenic/gene knockout animals where the animals can become susceptible to diseases where special conditions of maintenance are required due to the altered metabolic activities.

BIBLIOGRAPHY

1. Guidelines on the regulation of scientific experiments on animals, Ministry of Environment and Forest (Animal Welfare Division), Govt. of India, June 2007.

Section B

Clinical Pharmacology

- ➲ Drug Regulatory Bodies in India
- ➲ New Drug Development
- ➲ Institutional Ethics Committee
- ➲ Principle of ICH-GCP
- ➲ Investigators Responsibilities
- ➲ Protocol Writing
- ➲ Pharmacovigilance and PVPI
- ➲ Schedule Y
- ➲ Informed Consent

Drug Regulatory Bodies in India

Drug regulation is important to promote various activities to ensure the efficacy, safety and quality of drug. Every country has its own regulatory authority, which is responsible to enforce the rules and regulations and issue guidelines for drug development, licensing, registration, manufacturing, marketing and labeling of pharmaceutical products.

The drug regulation consists of:

1. Drug laws
2. Drug regulatory agencies
3. Drug regulatory boards
4. Quality control
5. Drug information centres

In order to regulate the import, manufacture, distribution and sale of drugs and cosmetics, the Drugs and Cosmetics Act, 1940 ('D&C Act') was introduced in India in 1940. Drugs and Health is in concurrent list of Indian Constitution. It is governed by both centre and state governments under the Drugs and Cosmetics Act, 1940.

MAIN REGULATORY BODIES IN INDIA

Ministry of Health and Family Welfare

Ministry	Regulatory bodies	Functional area
Ministry of Health and Family Welfare (MHFW)	Central Drug Standard Control Organization (CDSCO)	• Main drug licensing authority of India • Laying down standards
	Headed by	• Banning drugs and FDCs

Contd.

Ministry	Regulatory bodies	Functional area
	Drug Controller General of India (DCGI)	• Clinical trial related permission
Ministry of Science and Technology	Indian Council of Medical Research (ICMR)	• Formulate, coordinate and promote biomedical research and ethical principles
Ministry of Chemical and Petrochemicals	National Pharmaceutical Pricing Authority (NPPA)	• Decide ceiling price of drugs
Ministry of Commerce and Industry	Patent office CPCSEA	• Safeguard the patency of new drugs
Ministry of Environment and Forest	CPCSEA Genetic Engineering Approval Committee (GEAC)	• To promote the humane care of the animal used in biomedical research • Establishment of Institutional animal ethics committee (IAEC) • Control of biological-vaccines, antibodies, etc.

CDSCO

- In India, the Central Drugs Standard Control Organization (CDSCO) is the main regulatory body currently regulating import, sale and manufacture of medical devices which have been notified as drugs by virtue of Section 3(b) (IV) of the D&C Act.
- The CDSCO lays down standards of drugs, cosmetics, diagnostics and devices and issues licenses to drug manufacturers and importers.
- It also lays downregulatory measures, amendments to acts and rules and regulates market authorization of new drugs, clinical research in India and standards of imported drugs, etc.
- Headquartered in New Delhi, the CDSCO is India's main regulatory body for pharmaceuticals and medical devices and within the CDSCO, the Drug Controller General of India (DCGI) is responsible for the regulation of pharmaceuticals and medical devices.

- The DCGI is advised by the Drug Technical Advisory Board (DTAB) and the Drug Consultative Committee (DCC).
- Licensing and classification of medical devices are handled by the Central Licensing Approval Authority (CLAA).
- The CLAA is also responsible for setting and enforcing safety standards, appointing notified bodies to oversee conformity assessment, conducting post-market surveillance and issuing warnings and recalls for adverse events.

Functions

- Laying down standards of drugs, cosmetics, diagnostics and devices.
- Laying downregulatory measures, amendments to acts and rules.
- To regulate market authorization of new drugs.
- To regulate clinical research in India to approve licenses to manufacture certain categories of drugs as Central Licence Approving Authority, i.e. for blood banks, large volume parenteral and vaccines and sera.
- To regulate the standards of imported drugs.
- Work relating to the Drugs Technical Advisory Board (DTAB) and Drugs Consultative Committee (DCC). Testing of drugs by central drugs labs.
- Publication of Indian pharmacopoeia.

New Drug Development

INTRODUCTION

Process of drug development is broadly divided in 3 main phases

Drug discovery	2–5 years
Preclinical phase	1.5–2 years
Clinical trials	5–7 years
Application to regulatory authorities	1.5 years

Regulatory authority India—CDSCO, USA—US-FDA, UK—MHRA

Duration and Cost of Drug Development
Average time   10 –12 years.
Out of 10,000–30,000 potential substances
Only 1 could make it to the market
Cost: 500 million to 2,000 million USD.

DRUG DISCOVERY

Objectives of this phase is to find the lead compound and lead optimization.

Lead compound: Chemicals have potential to develop into new drug.

Lead optimization: Attempts are made to increase its potency at target site. Also made it pharmacokinetically better—find out 1 or 2 such compounds.

HIT: The drug molecule initially tried for developing into the drug is called HIT.

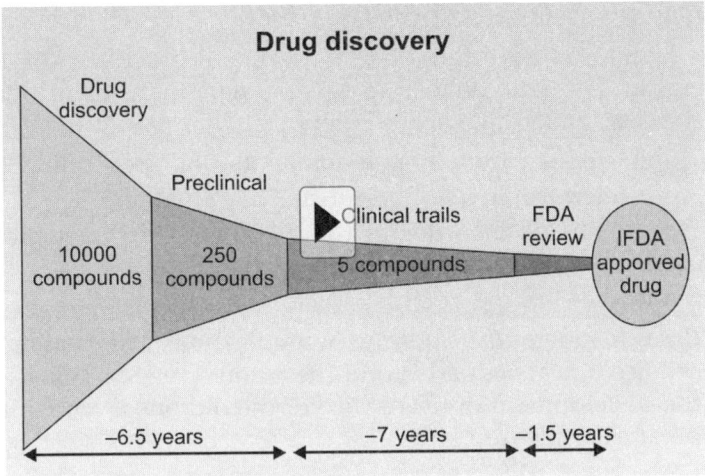

Fig. 12.1: Process of drug discovery

Various methods used to screen the biological and therapeutic activity of the compound are:

High throughput screening: To fast track the methods of drug development.

Quantitative structure activity relation (QSAR).

Combinatorial Chemistry

Various approaches used in this phase are:
• Random screening
• Serendipity
• Rational drug designing
• Drug metabolite—pro-drug/active metabolite

Random Screening

Major drugs in the pharmacology are discovered by this approach, i.e. morphine, atropine, digoxin, cyclosporine. This is a blind hitting procedure where new chemical entity is subjected to a battery of pharmacological screening procedures to explore different types of biological activity. The studies are conducted on animal models/isolated tissue. The major limitation of this method is that they are cumbersome, time consuming, expensive and may be fruitless.

Serendipity (Happy Observation/By Chance)

By chance observation of the therapeutic activity of the chemical. This later on lead to development in the drug. Some of the classic examples are as below:

Antibacterial activity of penicillin notatum—penicillin

Antibacterial activity of prontosil dye—sulfonamide

Haemorrhagic disorder in the cattle fed on sweet grass-warferin

Explosive—Nitroglycerin

Repositioning of the old drug: Serendipitious observation of pharmacological action beyond the primary effect. This leads to the development of newer use of the old one. Some of the popular examples are:

Drug	Older indication	Newer indication
Methotrexate	Anticancer	Psoriasis, rheumatoid arthritis
Lignocaine	Local anaesthetic	Antiarrhythmic
Phenytoin	Anticonvulsant	Antiarrhythmic
Cyclophosphamide, azathioprine	Anticancer	Immunosuppression
Retinoic acid	Acne	Leukemia
Bromocriptine	Parkinsonism	Diabetes mellitus
Amantadine	Antiviral	Antiparkinsonian
Ropinirole	Antiparkinsonian	Restless leg syndrome
Aspirin	Anti-inflammatory	Antiplatelet
Amphotericin B	Antifungal	Leishmaniasis
Bupropion	Depression	Smoking session
Topiramate	Anticonvulsant	Antiobesity
Liraglutide	Antidiabetic	Antiobesity
Gabapentine and pregabaline	Anticonvulsant	Neuropathic pain

Rational Drug Designing

This is most widely used method nowadays. This includes two different approaches depending upon target.

Compound centred approach

Pharmacological activity of the compound is explored by various methods like natural sources, synthetically made, alteration in chemical structure.

Natural: Insulin, iron, calcium, benzyl penicillin.

Purely synthetic: Aspirin, warferin.

Semisynthetic: Synthetically drug can be derived by *modification in the molecular structure (SAR)*: Semisynthetic penicillin—amoxycillin, piperacillin, cloxacillin.

Enantiomers: Nonsuperimposable mirror images of the molecule. Usually racemic mixture of the drug is used containing levo and dextoisomers. Later on it was found that pharmacological effect is because of only one component. While other can be toxic. Some of the examples are given below:

Drug	*Toxic effect*
Bupivacaine	R—bupivacaine—cardiotoxic
Thalidomide	s—Thalidomide—Phocomelia
Salbutamol	s—enantiomer is toxic
Ketamine	R—ketamine—abnormal muscle movement
L-dopa	Dextro is toxic

Pharmaceutical companies have overused this approach and this ended with *molecular manipulation*.

These are called 'me-too drugs' and ended with **drug explosion.** Examples: ACE inhibitors, ARBs, DPP 4 inhibitors, statins, H2 blockers, CCBs

Target centred approach

Depending upon the need in the therapy the biochemical structure like enzyme or biomolecular like receptor is made as the target.

Example: In hypertension—ACE inhibitors (ACE is target) and ARB—angiotensin II is target

Advantage: Easy lead compound and optimization

PRECLINICAL STUDIES

These are done on the experimental animal studies.

As per the biomedical ethics guidelines any new drug/new medical device is first tested on the animals first. These studies are conducted according to standards and code laid by GLP and schedule Y.

Various studies conducted in preclinical phase are:
- Pharmacodynamic studies
- Toxicological studies
- Special toxicity

Pharmacokinetic Studies

Promising compound after toxicological study: Assessment of safety index

Pharmacodynamic studies are conducted CO on whole animal/*in vivo* like dog, cat, guinea pig. For example, BIP, ECG, HR, CO. If the compound is promising further *in vitro*/isolated tissue at receptor level, vascular smooth muscles are done.

Toxicological Studies

These studies are done to determine the safety of drugs. These are done in at least two animal species and one should be rodent (its physiology matches with the human). These studies are done by two different routes, one of them should be for therapeutic use.

Various toxicological studies are as follows:
- Acute toxicity
- Subacute toxicity
- Chronic toxicity
- Special toxicity
- Reproductive toxicity
- Teratogenicity
- Carcinogenicity and mutagenicity
- Safety index.

Acute Toxicity

This test is done in two animal species and two different routes (proposed route).

LD50, i.e. dose lethal to 50% experimental animals is found out. In this test the single or multiple large doses of the drug is administered to the animal and the animal is observed for 7 to 14 days.

Subacute Toxicity

This is done in the two animal species and aim of the test is to find out the vulnerable organ for toxic effect. Maximum tolerated dose is given for 4 weeks–3 months. Biochemical, hematological changes are noted. Then the animal is sacrificed and histopathological changes are observed.

Chronic Toxicity

This is done if the drug is intended for chronic use, i.e. for 6–9 months. This is done in two animal species and one should be rodent.

Special Toxicity

US FDA has made it compulsory.

Reproductive Performance

This is done to assess the effect of drug on the reproductive function starting from reproductive behaviour, fertility to developmental and behavioral abnormalities in the offspring.

Mutagenicity/Genotoxicity

These studies are done to find out the adverse effect of drug on chromosome and genetic material.

Several *in vitro* and *in vivo* tests are done to assess genotoxic effect of the drug but most important is **Ame's test** done in *Salmonella typhi*.

Ame's Test

Salmonella typhimurium requires histidine for their growth. Drug which has potential to cause mutation will cause these organisms to grow without histidine.

Local Toxicity Studies

These are done when the drug is intended for local use like ocular–draisize test (rabbit), dermal test—guinea pig maximization test.

Safety Index

LD50/ED50, Therapeutic index—median lethal dose/median effective dose, (MTD)—maximum tolerated dose. In preclinical studies MTD is calculated which is later on interpolated to human depending upon body weight, surface area and other physiological parameters.

Investigational New Drug (IND) Application

Once the compound passes preclinical studies, an application is made to the related authorized drug control body—UK: CSM, USA: FDA, India: DCGI. This is to get the IND status for the molecule. One cannot start with the clinical trial till there is approval for IND.

CLINICAL TRIAL

It is systematic, ethical and prospective investigation in human subjects with the intention to discover, verify or compare the two or more drugs/medical device. Conducted in accordance with principles of Helsinki Declaration. It should be conducted in accordance with GCP (Good Clinical Practice) and other applicable regulatory guidelines.

Some important features of clinical trials are:

Designs

Parallel: Both the group will run parallel throughout the study period.

Crossover: The study population will be exposed to both the treatment option after washout period.

The advantage of the parallel design is it will be completed in short period. But it will require more number of patients and resources. In crossover the duration of trial will be longer but less number of study population will be required and the result will be more credential because of the constant endogenous factors. Sequential trial—where the matching study groups are taken (grade III breast cancer), this type of studies are done to hasten the study results. It is difficult to get patients.

Control/comparator: It can be placebo or the standard treatment option available.

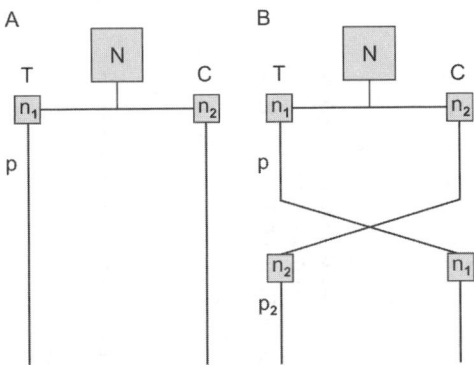

Fig. 12.2: Diagrammatic representation of parallel and crossover designs

Bias: Sometime the patient or the investigator can favour particular treatment group. This will create bias and credibility of the data will be reduced. Every participant should get an equal chance of selection in both the treatment group. This can be prevented by blinding and randomization.

Blinding: This is unaware of group.

• Single blind where investigator is unaware about the treatment option given to the subject.

• Double blind where both investigator and patient both are blinded.

Randomization: The treatment group is randomly allocated and the computer generated tables are used for this.

Specifying the inclusion and exclusion criteria are very important.

End point: Primary and secondary.

Sample size: Important to calculate an appropriate sample size so that a statistically significant result is found.

PHASES OF CLINICAL TRIALS

Phase zero : Micro-dosing
Phase I   : Human pharmacology and safety
Phase II   : Therapeutic exploration and dose ranging
Phase III   : Therapeutic confirmation/comparison
Phase IV   : Post-marketing

Phase Zero/Microdosing: This is new addition to the exploratory phase. The drug is administered in subtherapeutic/

Phases	Phase I *Human pharmacology and safety*	Phase II *Therapeutic exploration and dose ranging*	Phase III *Therapeutic confirmation/comparison*	Phase IV *Post-marketing surveillance/studies*
Objective	• Safety on first human use • Pharmacokinetic • Dose finding	• Efficacy, dose ranging • Detect—ADR	• Effectiveness on larger population • Compare with STD/placebo • Safety data	• Epidemiology • Rare ADR, drug interaction • Off label use/use pattern • Special population: Pregnancy, elderly paediatrics, risk benefit, co-morbidities
Participants	• Healthy volunteers	• Patients: Target disease	• Patients: Target disease	• Patients: Target disease
Number	• <100	• 100–500	• Up to 1000	• Community population
Setting	• ICU/24 hours monitoring	• IPD	• OPD/IPD	• OPD
Design	• Single centre, open label and control	• Usually single centre, blinded, placebo or active control, strict inclusion criteria	• Multicentre, blinded, randomised, control • Less strict inclusion criteria	• Community study
Duration	• Few days to month	• Few months to 1 year	• 1–5 years	• NDS: First 4 years • PSUR: Very 6 monthly –2 years

microdose in healthy volunteers. In small number, i.e. 10–15. This is first testing of drug in the human. 1/100th effective dose is administered to the human to find out the pharmacokinetic and pharmacodynamic data. This phase dose not give any data on safety and efficacy of the drug. This phase hasten the process of clinical trial and the cost is also reduced. This is still not mandatory.

BIBLIOGRAPHY

1. HL Sharma and KK Sharma, Principles of Pharmacology, 2nd edition 2011, Paras Publication, Chapter No. 8, Drug Discovery and Clinical Evaluation of New Drugs.
2. S Parasuraman. Toxicological screening. J pharmacol Pharmacother, 2011. Apr–Jun; 2(2):74–79.

Institutional
Ethics Committee

In biomedical research (clinical trial and related research work) ethics, i.e. moral principles should be followed. This should be applicable from beginning of the research work till its end. To ensure the rights, safety and well-being of human subjects, several laws and guidelines have been formulated. This responsibility is taken care by independent ethics (IEC) committee/IRB (institutional review board). It is now mandatory to seek approval of the study protocol from registered independent ethics committee before the study is initiated.

INDEPENDENT ETHICS COMMITTEE

This is permitted to review the protocol for bioavailability and bioequivalence studies. As per the newer amendments, these committees are permitted to review the protocol for clinical trial, if it is associated with hospital which is within 50 km.

Several milestone in the history of biomedical research because of non-ethical issues.

1. **Nuremberg's code (1947):** It was formulated at the time of Word War II followed by the inhuman experiment conducted on the prisoners. It has led down the rules for permissible medical experiments in humans.
2. **Declaration of Helsinki (1967):** In Germany in 1964 thalidomide was used widely in pregnant female as an antiemetic for morning sickness. It led to serious congenital malformation in the offspring (seal limb). The drug was

marked without preclinical studies on the rodent. This is known as Thalidomide tragedy. This has brought about the concept of Inform consent, ethics committee approval, vulnerable population and importance of standard as comparator.

3. **Belmont report (1979):** Tuskegee trial syphilis trial conducted by Nazi doctors on the prisoners. They were deprived of the medication to study the disease process. To avoid the injustice with study participation The National Commission wrote the Belmonte report "Ethical principles and guidelines for the protection of Human rights". Three fundamental principles of this report were respect, beneficence and justice for the study participants.

4. **Indian version of GCP:** Guidelines were issued by CSDCO in 2001.

5. **ICMR:** Ethical guidelines for biomedical research in human subject. First formed in 2006 and regularly updated, latest is in 2017.

6. **Schedule Y formulated in 2005:** Guidelines for conduct of clinical trial for new drug, import and export of new drug.

7. **As per the recent updates:** It is mandatory to take ethics committee approval.

Composition

At least 7 members form the committee, medical, paramedical, legal and community representative. Chairperson—outside the institute, member secretory, medical scientist/pharmacologist, clinician/subject expert, legal expert, social scientist/ethicist, lay person. Quoram is formed by at least last 5.

Responsibilities

1. To safeguard the rights, safety and well-being of the participants in the clinical trial.

2. Review and approve the clinical trial protocol. In case IEC revokes the approval, decision should be communicated to the investigator and regulatory authority.

3. Review of the documentation furnished by investigator—protocol, investigator's brochure, case record form (CRF), informed consent form (ICF) and patient information sheet

(PIS), investigator's CV, information about payments and compensation available to subjects, scientific literature about the product.

4. Record and documents should be retain for at least 5 years after completion of study.
5. **Periodic review of the site of on-going clinical trial:** To ensure SOPs and protocol are being followed.
6. To conduct meeting and keep record of the meeting.
7. Risk vs benefit assessment of the study
8. SAE reporting to the regulatory authority within 30 calendar days.
9. Special attention should be paid to trials that may include vulnerable subjects.
10. **Non-therapeutic trial:** Ethical concerns should be adequately addressed and should meet applicable regulatory requirements for such trials.

BIBLIOGRAPHY

1. http://icmr.nic.in/ethical.pdf
2. http://ohsr.od.nih.gov/guidelines/nuremberg.html
3. Schedule Y 1995, Amendments, 2013, CSDCO

14

Principle of ICH-GCP

International conference on harmonization (ICH) of technical requirements for registration of pharmaceuticals for human use.

It is a supra regional body comprising of:

Primary participants: USA, Europe and Japan

Observers: Canada, Australia and Scandinavian countries

In 1996, ICH-GCP guidelines were formed keeping in mind the following principles.

Milestones: Before 20th century there was no regulation for conduct of clinical trial.

It deals with the following aspects of clinical trials:

Q: Quality, S: Safety, E: efficacy, M: multidisciplinary

E6 guidelines: Describe the principles of efficacy

Indian version of GCP: Guidelines were issued by CSDCO in 2001.

GCP (good clinical practice): A standard for the design, conduct, performance, monitoring, auditing, recording, analysis and reporting of clinical trial.

Objectives

• It provides assurance that all data and reported results are credible and accurate.

• The rights, integrity and confidentiality of trial subject are protected.

These principles are applicable for:

1. All clinical trials (drug devices, procedures)
2. Bioavailability and bioequivalence study
3. All epidemiological studies.

Principles

1. Clinical trials should be conducted in accordance with the ethical principles of Declaration of Helsinki, GCP and applicable regulatory requirement(s).
2. Risk vs benefit ratio should be in favour of the study individual trial subject and society.
3. Priority should be given for the protection of rights, safety, and well-being of the trial subjects over interests of science and society.
4. The available nonclinical and clinical data on an investigational product should be adequate to support the proposed clinical trial.
5. Clinical trials should be scientifically sound and conducted in accordance with the predesigned study protocol.
6. A trial should be conducted after taking the favourable approval from independent ethics committee.
7. The medical care and decisions to the subject should be given by qualified physician/qualified dentist.
8. Each individual involved in conducting a trial should be qualified by education, training, and experience.
9. Voluntary informed consent should be obtained from every subject prior to clinical trial participation.
10. All the clinical data should be recorded and stored accurately.
11. The confidentiality of records and study participants should be protected.
12. Investigational products should be manufactured, handled, and stored in accordance with good manufacturing practice (GMP) and should be administered as the protocol.
13. All SOPs should be designed prior to the conduct to assure the quality of clinical trial.

BIBLIOGRAPHY

1. Wendy Boyachuk; Ball G. Conducting GCP-compliant clinical research. John Wiley and Sons, 1999.

Investigators Responsibilities

1. **Investigator's qualifications and agreements:**
   - The investigator(s) should be qualified by education, training, and experience.
   - All the qualifications specified by the applicable regulatory requirement(s), and should provide evidence of such qualifications.
   - He/she should be thoroughly familiar with the appropriate use of the investigational product(s).
   - He/she should permit monitoring by the sponsor, and inspection by the appropriate regulatory authority.
   - Maintain a list of appropriately qualified persons to whom the investigator has delegated significant trial-related duties.
2. **Adequate resources:** He/she should be able to recruit the required number of suitable subjects within the specific period.
3. He/she should be able to complete the trial within the agreed trial period. He/she should adequately informed about the protocol, the investigational product(s), and their trial-related duties and functions to all persons assisting with the trial.
4. **Medical care of trial subjects:** Responsible for all trial-related medical (or dental) decisions including management of adverse drug reaction.
5. He/she should try to find out the reason for premature withdrawl of the participant.

6. **Communication with IRB/IEC:** Before initiating a trial, the investigator/institution should seek written and dated approval/favourable opinion from the IEC. During the trial the investigator/institution should provide to the IRB/IEC all documents subject to review.

7. **Compliance with protocol:** Should conduct the trial in compliance with the protocol agreed by the sponsor, IEC and regulatory authority.

8. **Deviation with protocol:** Any deviation from the approved protocol should be documented and reported to the IEC, sponsor and regulatory authority with suitable explanation.

9. **Investigator product:** Procurement, record of delivery dates, quantity, batch no, expiry dates and unique code number assign to IP and trial subject, doses and record of storage.

10. **Randomization procedures and unblinding:** Should follow the trial's randomization procedures. Decoding should be done only in accordance with the protocol. Premature unblinding which could be accidental or due to a serious adverse event should be promptly reported and documented to the sponsor.

11. **Informed consent of trial subjects:** Informed consent should be taken according to the guideline of GCP and Declaration of Helsinki. Should have the favourable opinion approval of the written informed consent form. Details are given in the IEC chapter.

12. **Records and reports:** The investigator should ensure the accuracy, completeness, legibility, and timeliness of the data. Source documents are the one from which all data is captured, i.e. discharge card, prescription, investigation. All information of all the original records of clinical findings, observation and certified copies of investigations are necessary for reconstruction and evaluation of clinical trial. Essential documents are those that individually and collectively permit evaluation of conduct of clinical trial and quality of data generated, i.e. CRF, ICF. Data reported on the CRF, that are derived from source documents, should be consistent with the source documents or the

discrepancies should be explained. Essential documents should be retained until at least 5 years after the last approval of a marketing application.

13. **Progress reports:** The investigator should submit written trial status to the IEC annually. If requested more frequently by IEC.

14. **Safety reporting:** All serious adverse events should be reported immediately to the sponsor, IEC, head of the institution and regulatory authorities (within 24 hours).

15. **Premature termination or suspension of a trial:** In case of prematurely terminated or suspended for any reason should promptly inform to the trial subjects and assure appropriate therapy and follow-up for them.

16. **Final report by investigator:** At the end of the trial should inform the IEC, sponsor, head of the institution about the trial outcome.

BIBLIOGRAPHY

1. ICH Topic E6.Note for guidance on good clinical practice, CPMP/ICH/135/95.

Protocol Writing

Protocol is defined as a document that describes the background, rationale, objective, design, methodology, statistical considerations and organization of a trial. It describes the details about how the trial is to be conducted and scientific rationale for the structure of a research project. It is a written agreement between the investigator, participant and the scientific community.

A typical protocol has the following elements—title page, signature page, background information, objectives, study design, study population, study procedures, statistical considerations, subject confidentiality, informed consent process, literature references, supplements/appendices.

COMPLETE PROTOCOL

Adequate details required for the reader to understand requirement for the study, i.e. details about blood pressure measurement procedure in the antihypertensive study.

As per current CDSCO guidelines it is mandatory to register all the clinical trial with CTRI (Clinical Trial Registry of India) and should obtained a registration number.

1. **Title page:** It obtains the document and should contain following details about the study: Study title, protocol number, sponsor, and author to the reader. It should also contain the protocol title, protocol identifying number and date, if any amendment—amendment number and date along with the version number, whether it is final or draft

and date of this version, name and address of the sponsor and monitor, name and title of the person(s) authorized to sign the protocol and the protocol amendment(s) for the sponsor, name, title, address and telephone number(s) of the sponsors medical expert, name and title of the investigator(s) who is responsible for conducting the trial and address and telephone number(s) of trial site(s), name, title, address and telephone number(s) of the qualified physician, name and address of the clinical laboratory and other medical department or institutions involved. Full title should include the summary study design, medicinal products, nature of the treatment, comparator, placebo, indication, patient population, setting (e.g. inpatient, outpatient), randomized, double blind, multiple studies.

2. **Signature page:** Should include contact details of participating site, sponsor and sponsor's medical advisor if not already given above.

3. **Content page:** Helps navigation through the document by a large number of different people that will be needed throughout the life of the trial.

4. **List of abbreviations:** All abbreviations should be listed and defined. Accepted international medical abbreviations should be used. Project specific abbreviations should be standardized within each project.

5. **Compliance statement:** The protocol should include a statement that the trial will be conducted in compliance with the protocol, good clinical practice (GCP) and the applicable regulatory requirements.

6. **Protocol summary/synopsis:** This summary should be only one to two pages long. It should give the reader information to understand the rationale for the trial, its objectives and the methods that will be used to achieve the objective.

7. **Background information:** Should contain the name and description of the investigational product, summary of findings from nonclinical studies, summary of the known and potential risks and if any, to human subjects, description and justification for the route of administration, dosage, dosage regimen and treatment period, it should be able to justify the need of the study.

8. **Study objective/aims**
   - A clinical trial often has both primary and secondary objectives, and these should be identified as such in the protocol.
   - *Study end-points:* It is beneficial if the parameters chosen can demonstrate end-points related to reduced progression or reversal of disease, improved quality of life, reduced mortality, improved symptomatology of patient, etc.
   - *Study rationale*: It defines the need for conducting the study.

9. **Study design:** Trial design is responsible for scientific integrity and credibility of data generated from clinical trial.

   Various factors which should be considered while selecting the study designing are choice of control group, methods used for avoiding bias like blinding, randomization, explanation for crossover design, financial resources available, rationale for selection of particular trial designing.

   Examples of study designs: Double blind, case control, cohort, cross-sectional, nested case control, double dummy or hybrid designs.

10. **Randomization:** This is the technique used for getting an equal chance for section of treatment group. Computer generated randomization table is used for this. The mode of randomization should be specified in the protocol.

11. **Inclusion and exclusion criteria:** Inclusion criteria constitute the definition of patient characteristics required for entry into clinical trial. One needs to consider the narrow and broad limits for identifying the specific inclusion and exclusion criteria.

    Narrow vs broad limits: Excessive broad criteria can result in the recruitment of heterogeneous group of people and interpretation and relevance of the trial will be questioned. Too narrow inclusion criteria can create difficulty in getting adequate sample size. Data generated from this population will not be applicable to general population. Advantage of narrow criteria will be entry of homogenous population and hence meaningful data and interpretation.

Various inclusion criteria are:

- *Demographic criteria of the patients:* Age, sex, race, weight, socioeconomic status, pregnancy, lactation, tobacco, alcohol hypersensitive to study medication, non-medicine allergies, emotional limitations
- *Characteristics of disease and treatment:* Disease which is under evaluation, concomitant medication, comorbid condition, previous hospitalization, operation and procedure.
- *Environmental and other factors:* Participation in another clinical trial, other part of same trial, any other trial using same medicine.

12. **Screening:** A screening is an evaluation of potential patients to determine their eligibility to enter a clinical trial. It is based on an interview or review of medical records. In prospective clinical trial evaluation test like physical, laboratory. It may be done in steps. The screening procedure should be elaborated in study protocol.

13. **Recruitment:** Procedure for recruitment of the study participants should be mentioned in the protocol, e.g. advertisement, pamphlets, etc.

14. **Sample size:** The number of patients required for a clinical trial refers to the number of patients who finish a trial rather than the number who enter.

A false positive result may occur in all trials, the chances are higher when fewer patients are enrolled. Numerous biases and errors in a clinical trial may be minimized by increasing the number of patients entered until adequate power is obtained. Pilot study with small sample size is conducted to obtain the information and feasibility of study.

15. **Statistics:** Statistical methods which will be used for analysis of primary and secondary end points should be included. Timing of interim analysis should be included. Level of significance and its relation with clinical significance should be mentioned. Any deviation from mentioned statistical methodology should be reported.

16. **Criteria for termination of clinical trial:** Specifically for early termination of trial. Placebo arm in case of life-threatening disease.

17. **Treatment schedules:** All details of the treatment including test group and control group should be mentioned. This includes name, dosage, frequency, duration, follow-up, special instructions. In case of study medication: Source, storage, in case of reconstitution: Procedure, name of the supplier. How the patient will be treated after study period, including study medication supply. Details of the treatment in case of serious adverse drug reaction, also decoding in this case.

18. **Concomitant treatment/rescue medication:** Medicine which should be taken and which should not be taken should be mentioned in the protocol. This requires careful evaluation to avoid drug interaction with the study medication. Rescue medication can be standardized for particular trial.

19. **Compliance of study participants:** Various methods which can be used to ensure the compliance of study participants are—pill count, subject's diary, feedback from relative, return of packaging material, watching subject swallow the pill, observing the pill in oral cavity.

20. **Number of evaluations/visits:** Number of visits during study period should be mentioned in the protocol. Usually factors affecting number of visits differ with the trial. In general, number of visits is more in the initial part of trial than in the later period. A thought should be given to cost of money, energy, time and the data generated from the visit. Usually it is in multiples like every 2 weeks for 3 visit followed by every 4 weeks for remaining.

21. **Post-treatment period:** Evaluation in this period is mainly to evaluate withdrawal effects and ensure patient safety.

22. **Access to source data/documents:** Sponsors, trial related monitoring authority, auditing body and regulatory authority.

23. **Quality control and quality assurance:** It should be according to GCP, GLP and GMP guidelines.

24. **Ethics—certain ethical issues are necessary to address**
    1. Screening and recruitment of patient
    2. Providing information to referring physician
    3. Protocol violation
    4. Special consideration given to vulnerable population.

25. **Protocol violation:** Sponsor and investigator should be sensitive for protocol violation. Minor deviations may not raise sensitive issues.

BIBLIOGRAPHY

1. Bolla M, et al EORTC guidelines for writing protocols for clinical trials for radiotherapy. Radiotheroncol 1995;36(1):1–8.
2. Mahmoud F. Fathalla. WHO regional publications eastern mediterranen series 30, a practical guide for health researcher, 2004.

Pharmacovigilance and PVPI

This was derived from the Greek word "pharmakon" meaning a drug or medicine and from the Latin word "vigilans" meaning watchful or careful.

World Health Organization defines pharmacovigilance as "The science and activities related to the detection, assessment, understanding and prevention of adverse effects or any other drug related problem."

Certain important definitions:

Adverse drug reaction (ADR): These are the noxious and unintended effects of the drug and which occurs at doses normally used in humans for their prophylaxis, diagnosis or therapy of disease or for the modification of physiological function.

Adverse event (AE): Any untoward medical occurrence that may occur during treatment with a pharmaceutical product but which does not necessarily have a causal relationship with the treatment.

Serious Adverse Event (SAE): A serious adverse event or reaction is any untoward medical occurrence that at any dose:
- Results in death
- Life threatening
- Requires hospitalization/prolongation of existing hospitalization
- Results in persistent/significant disability/incapacity
- Leads to congenital anomaly

CLASSIFICATION OF ADR

Type	Type of effect	Example
Type A	Augmented	Insulin—hypoglycaemia
		B-blocker—bradycardia
Type B	Bizzare	Penicillin—anaphylaxis
		Anticonvulsants—hypersensitivity
Type C	Chronic	NSAIDs-induced ulcers
		Corticosteroids-induced osteoporosis
Type D	Delayed	Chemotherapy—secondary malignancy
Type E	End of treatment	Phenytoin—withdrawal seizures
		Clonidine withdrawal—rebound
		hypertension
Type F	Failure of therapy	Failure of contraception

NEED FOR PHARMACOVIGILANCE

1. Unreliability of pre-clinical safety data
2. Rare side effect is not detected during preclinical and clinical trial, e.g. clozapine induced agranulocytosis.
3. Early detection of newer/unknown.
4. Changing pharmaceutical marketing strategies, i.e. aggressive marketing.
5. Changing physician's and patient's preferences
   - Increasing use of newer drugs.
   - Increasing use of drugs to improve quality of life.
   - Shift of supervised to self-administered therapy.

AIM OF PHARMACOVIGILANCE

- Expand precaution for patient.
- Increase public protection from the new products.
- To contribute the knowledge of value, detriment, efficiency and hazard of medicines.
- Endorse healthy communication to the community.
- To promote rational and safe use of medicines.

PHARMACOVIGILANCE/ADR MONITORING METHODS

As per International Conference on Harmonization (ICH), methods can be divided into two types depending on the way of reporting:

Passive surveillance: It encompasses all spontaneous adverse effects reported from hospitals and patients.

- *Spontaneous reporting system (SRS):* Healthcare workers like physician, nurses, pharmacist, pharmaceutical manufacturers.
- *Case series:* Presenting series of case report containing the ADR of interest.
- *Stimulated reporting:* Online reporting of adverse events and methodical motivation of reporting based on predesigned method.

Active surveillance: This method try to find out the ADR and events in number by constant pre-organized process. This method provides a complete information on large scale.

- *Sentinel sites:* It is done by revising medical records or questioning patients/physicians to collect the data on reported ADR from these sites, e.g. government hospital.
- *Drug event monitoring:* In this method the event is traced to do the data generation. Electronic/automated health insurance claims are used as a source.
- *Registries:* List of patients maintained according to disease or exposure, e.g. blood dyscrasias, cutaneous reactions, congenital malformations.

A few other methods are: Comparative observational studies, cross-sectional study, case-control study, cohort study, targeted clinical investigations, descriptive studies, natural history of disease, drug utilization study.

SRS (Spontaneous reporting system): The most important system for pharmacovigilance is spontaneous reporting system. This is oldest, most productive and cost-effective method of ADR reporting. The SRS involves the voluntary participation of health professionals, pharmacists, nurses and patients themselves for reporting the observations related to ADR.

PHARMACOVIGILANCE PROGRAM OF INDIA (PVPI)

History

In India, Central Drugs Standard Control Organization (CDSCO), Ministry of Health and Family Welfare, Government of India, launched the National Pharmacovigilance Programme (NPP) in November 2004. This was renamed PVPI in 2010.

Goals
- To ensure that the benefits of use of medicine outweighs the risks.
- Safeguard the health of the Indian population.

Aims
- To monitor adverse drug reactions (ADRs) in Indian population.
- To create awareness amongst health care professionals about the importance of ADR reporting in India.
- To monitor benefit—risk profile of medicines.
- Generate independent, evidence-based recommendations on the safety of medicines.
- Support the CDSCO for formulating safety related regulatory decisions for medicines.
- Communicate findings with all key stakeholders.
- Create a national centre of excellence at par with global drug safety monitoring standards.

Objectives
The program has three broad objectives:
- The short-term objective is to foster a reporting culture amongst the healthcare providers.

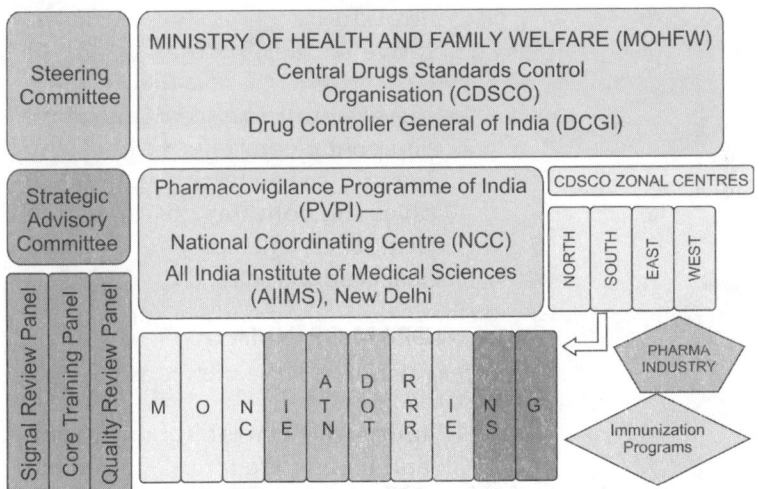

Fig. 17.1: Governance structure of PVPI

TABLE 17.1: Functions of the stakeholders

PVPI ADR monitoring centre in medical college (PVPI AMCs)	• Collection of ADR reports. • Perform follow up with the complainant to check completeness as per SOPs. • Data entry into vigiflow. • Reporting to PVPI National Coordinating Centre (PVPI NCC) through vigiflow. • Training/sensitization/feedback to physicians through newsletters circulated by the PVPI NCC.
PVPI ADR monitoring centre other than medical colleges [corporate hospitals, autonomous institutes, public health programmes]	• Collection of ADR reports. • Perform follow up with the complainant to check completeness as per SOPs. • Report the data to CDSCO HQ.
PVPI National Coordinating Centre (PVPI NCC, AIIMS, New Delhi)	• Preparation of SOPs, guidance documents and training manuals. • Data collation, cross-check completeness, causality assessment, etc as per SOPs. • Conduct training workshops of all enrolled centres. • Publication of medicines safety newsletter. • Reporting to CDSCO headquarters. • Analysis of the PMS, PSUR, AEFI data received from CDSCO HQ.
Zonal/Subzonal CDSCO offices	• Provide procurement, financial and administrative support to ADR monitoring centres. • Report to CDSCO HQ.
CDSCO, HQ, New Delhi	• Take appropriate regulatory decision and actions on the basis of recommendations of PVPI NCC–AIIMS. • Propagation of medicine safety related decisions to stakeholders. • Collaboration with WHO—Uppsala Monitoring Centre—Sweden. • Provide for budgetary provisions and administrative support to run national PVPI.

- The intermediate objective is to involve a large number of healthcare professionals for reporting and spread of information.
- The long-term objective of this program is to be a benchmark for global drug monitoring.

UMC

Uppasala monitoring center (UMC) located in Sweden is the global collaborating center.

Database where all the global data is stored is 'Vigibase'.

Software used for the recording is 'Vigiflow'.

Under this programme:

- The country is divided into zones and regions for operational convenience
- At the top: CDSCO (Central Drug Standard Control organization), New Delhi.

Followed by that

Two zonal pharmacovigilance centres

- Seth GS Medical College, Mumbai for South-West Zone.
- All India Institute of Medical Sciences (AIIMS), New Delhi —North-East Zone.

There are nine regional pharmacovigilance centres located:

1. Kolkata: Institute of Postgraduate Medical Education and Research—Seth Sukhlal Karnani Memorial (IPGMER—SSKM) Hospital.
2. Mumbai (TN Medical College and BYL Nair Charitable Hospital)
3. Nagpur (Indira Gandhi Medical College)
4. Pondicherry: Jawaharlal Insitute of Postgraduate Medical Education and Research (JIPMER).
5. NIZAMS—Hyderabad
6. BJMC—Ahmedabad
7. AIIMS—Bhopal
8. JSS—Medical college, Mysore
9. PGIMER—Chandigadh

Flowchart 17.1: Flow of ADR reporting to WHO

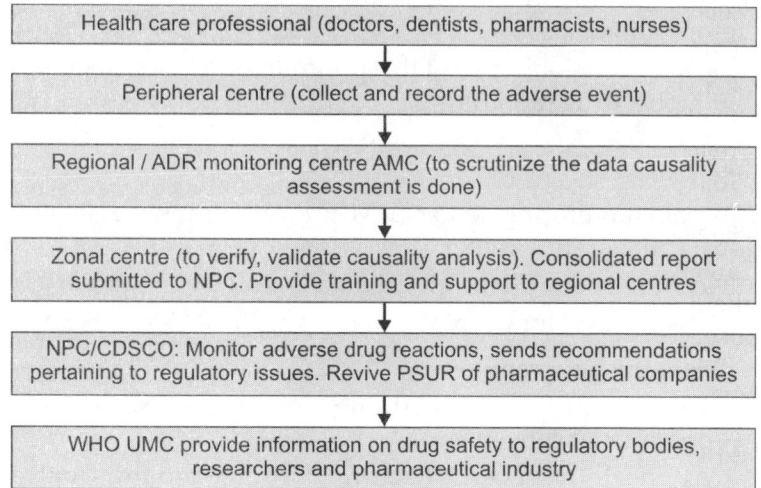

INDIVIDUAL CASE SAFETY REPORTS (ICSRs)

INDIVIDUAL CASE SAFETY REPORTS (ICSRs)

ICSRs are collected in predesigned suspected ADR reporting form, broadly consists of 4 sectors—patients information, suspected ADR, suspected medication and reporters information as shown in Flowchart 17.1.

Roles of Pharmacovigilance Programme of India

The purpose of the program is:
• To collect and analyse the reported data
• To reach to the conclusion

Thereby recommend the regulatory interventions for safeguarding the health of Indian population.

Recommendations can be:
  • Changing the composition
  • Black box warning
  • *Banning of particular drug:* In severe cases
  • *Prescription only drug:* To be sold only as POM

Example: Phenylpropanolamine, it was an ingredient of cough syrup (decongestant).

It was associated with haemorrhagic stroke in young females. US-FDA has taken the action of removing the content.

Provide the better understanding of ADR and factors affecting

Process in Pharmacovigilance

- Collect and record of AEs / ADRs
- Causality assessment and analysis of ADRs
- Collate and code in database: •WHO-ART (Adverse drug reaction terminology) and in MedDRA (Medical dictionary for regulatory activities)

Causality Assessment

Causality assessment is defined as the evaluation of the likelihood that a medicine was the causative agent of an observed adverse reaction.

It is done by using different logarithms: Narango's scale and WHO UMC scale.

WHO causality assessment	
Causality term	*Assessment criteria*
Certain	• Event or lab test abnormality with plausible time relationship to drug intake. • Cannot be explained by disease or other drugs. • Response to withdrawal plausible. • Event definitive pharmacologically. • Rechallenge satisfactorily, if necessary.
Probable/likely	• Event or lab test abnormality with reasonable time relationship to drug intake. • Unlikely to be attributed to disease or other drugs. • Response to withdrawal reasonable. • Rechallenge not required.
Possible	• Event or lab test abnormality with reasonable time relationship to drug intake. • Could also be explained by disease or other drugs. • Information on drug withdrawal lacking or unclear.
Unlikely	• Event/lab test abnormality, with a time to drug intake that makes a relationship improbable. • Disease or other drugs provide plausible explanation.
Conditional/ unclassified	• Event/lab test abnormality. • More data for proper assessment needed.
Un-assessable/ unclassified	• Report suggesting an adverse reaction. • Cannot be judged because information is insufficient or contradictory. • Data cannot be supplemented or verified.

Compute Risk: Benefit and Suggest Regulatory Action

- **Generate signal:** A signal is defined as reported information on a possible causal between an adverse event and a drug, the relationship being unknown or incompletely documented previously.
- **Periodic Safety Update Report (PSUR):** Periodic safety monitoring of the drug. All new drugs when comes into the market, they are sold as a status of *new drug* for four years.
- Manufacturing company is supposed to report the data to the concern regulatory authorities for four years.
- It is done as every 6 months for first 2 years followed by annually for 2 years.
- **Scope of PVPI:** Now it has extended to cover the safety data from blood and blood product related ADR under the HVPI —Haemovigilance Programme of India, launched in 2012 and headquarter in National Institute of Biologicals, Noida. Separate ADR reporting forms are available.
- **Materiovigilance programme of India (MVPI):** This deals with the collection of safety data on medical devices.

Schedule Y

- It is extension of Drugs and Cosmetic Act (DCA) 1940 and rules 1945. It gives "Requirements and guidelines for permission to import and/or manufacture of new drugs for sale or undertake clinical trials."
- It comprises the following rule
  - 122 A—Permission to import new drug
  - 122B—Manufacturing of new drug
  - 122 D—Import or manufacture FDC
  - 122DA—To conduct new drugs
  - 122 DD—Registration of ethics committee
  - 122 DAA—Definition of clinical trial
  - 122 DAB—Compensation
- Schedule Y was formulated by CDSCO (Central Drug Standards Control and Organisation) in 2005.

Salient Features of Schedule "Y"

- Application for permission to import or manufacture new drugs for sale or to undertake clinical trials shall be made in Form 44.
- Phase III trials are required to be conducted in India before permission to market the drug in India is granted.
- Following documents are required to submit along with the application for conduct of clinical trial except trial for life threatening/serious diseases or diseases of special relevance to the Indian health scenario.
- Investigator's brochure, proposed protocol, case record form, informed consent document(s), investigator's undertaking

and ethics committee clearance. Preclinical trial data and toxicological data. This can be omitted or concised in the trial of drug.

- Details about the responsibilities and role of sponsor, investigator and IEC.
- Conduct and specification of various phases of clinical trials (Phase 0–phase IV). Submission of periodic safety update report (PSUR) data by pharmaceutical companies for every new drug.
- Specification for conduct of preclinical toxicity studies: LD 50 should be done in two rodent species.
- Guidelines for conduct of clinical trial in special/vulnerable population: Geriatric, paediatrics, pregnancy and lactation, disabled.
- Guidelines for BA/BE studies.
- Rules for FDC approval
- Amendments are made in schedule "Y" on regular basis as per the need. Latest amendments are given as follows:
- 2005: Approval from ethics committee for clinical trial protocol is mandatory before start of the trial.
- 2013: Expansion of responsibilities of sponsor, investigator and ethics committee. This was in the form of specific period is given for reporting of SAE
- PI to DCGI, sponsor and ethics committee within 24 hours (SAE-death), non-death SAE—within 14 calendar days from the time of occurrence.
- Ethics committee to DCGI: All SAE (death and non-death SAE) within 30 calendar days.
- Sponsor to DCGI, EC and head of the institution—within 14 calendar days.
- Sponsor has to pay the compensation within 30 calendar days. This is order from DCGI.

Clinical Trial Related Injury

Any injury or death of the subject occurring in clinical trial due to following conditions will be considered clinical trial related injury and subject/his/her nominee are entitled for financial compensation.

1. Adverse effects of investigational product.
2. Violation from approved protocol, scientific misconduct or negligence by the investigator.
3. Failure of an investigational product to provide attended therapeutic effect.
4. Administration of placebo providing no therapeutic benefits.
5. Adverse effect due to concomitant medication.
6. Compensation for injury to a child *in utero* because of the participation of parent in clinical trial.
7. Injury due to any clinical trial procedure.

COMPENSATION IN CASE OF SAE

Compensation is calculated as follows:
- Quantum of compensation for SAE/Death = $B*F*R/99.37$
  where B = 8 Lakhs

  F = value from age table

  R = risk factor ranging from 0.5 to 4 depending on duration and severity of disease.
- Quantum of compensation for disability = 90% of death compensation × percentage disability
- Quantum of compensation for other SAE = $2*W*N$
  where W = minimum daily wage of an unskilled worker in Delhi

  N = No. of days of hospitalization

Informed Consent

A process by which a subject voluntarily confirms his or her willingness to participate in a particular trial, after having been informed of all aspects of the trial that are relevant to the subject's decision to participate. Informed consent is documented by means of a written, signed and dated informed consent form.

The goal of the informed consent process is to provide people with sufficient information so they can make informed choices about whether to begin or continue participation in clinical research.

Required components of patient information sheet (in patient's vernacular language)

1. Nature and purpose of study stating it as research.
2. Duration of participation with number of participants.
3. Procedures to be followed (route, number, time, food to be avoided, contraceptive intake).
4. Investigators details.
5. Investigations, if any, to be performed (blood withdrawl, USG, X-ray).
6. Foreseeable risks and discomforts adequately described and whether project involves more than minimal risk.
7. Benefits to participant, community or medical profession as may be applicable.
8. Alternative treatments, if available.
9. Steps taken for ensuring confidentiality.
10. Policy on compensation in trial related injury.

11. Complete voluntary participation and free to withdraw at any time.
12. Information about publication of data including photographs.
13. Post-trial access: Information regarding post-trial access of the drug and other intervention should be given to the study subjects.

Informed Consent Form (Patient's Vernacular Language)

1. Research title
2. It contains the patient details like name, age, gender, address.
3. Statements to ensure that patient has read and understood the content of the PIS.
4. Signature and thumb impression of the participant with date and place.
5. Investigators details
6. New addition to the ICF—occupation of the participants, income and name of the nominee in case of clinical trial related injury.
7. If the participant is minor (age 7–18 years), LAR (legally acceptable representative)/assent should be taken.

USUALLY A GUARDIAN

Waiver of Consent

1. When it is impractical to conduct research since confidentiality of personally identifiable information has to be maintained throughout research, e.g. study on disease burden of HIV/AIDS.
2. Emergency situations, when surrogate consent unavailable
3. Research on anonymised biological samples from deceased individuals, left over samples, cell lines, etc.
4. Research on publicly available information, documents, records, works, performances, reviews, etc.

Assent

'Assent' means a child's affirmative agreement to participate in research.

"All paediatric participants should be informed to the fullest extent possible about the study in a language and in terms that they are able to understand."—Schedule Y

Audio-Visual Consent

It was made mandatory for all clinical trials to obtain audio-visual consent from each study participant but now limited to only vulnerable population.

Section C
Biostatistics

- ➲ Data and Types of Data
- ➲ Hypothesis Testing
- ➲ Statistical Tests

Data and Types of Data

Statistics is the science of data analysis. Statistics allow generalisation of study results. It is important in human research because:

1. Enormous biological variability
2. Inability to control all confounding variables
3. Small differences are difficult to detect

Biostatistics: It is the study of statistical processes and method applied to collection, analysis and interpretation of biological data.

DATA

They are the values of measurement. Data can be divided into two categories, i.e. qualitative (counts) and quantitative (measurements).

Data Types

1. **Quantitative/neumeric/metric:** Values come from measurements using specific tools. This is further classified as discrete and continuous.
   - *Discrete:* Whole numbers, e.g. blood pressure—140/80 mmHg.
   - *Continuous*: Can take decimal places, e.g. height— 160.2 cm
2. **Qualitative/categorical:** Not measured by specific tools, e.g. colour, gender. This is further classified as nominal and ordinal.

- *Nominal:* Only names, e.g. colour, gender. Each value has equal importance.
- *Ordinal*: Some hierarchy is present, e.g. severity of pain: Mild, moderate, severe (VAS scale)

Data is also classified according to the following categories:

1. **Binary/dichotomous**, e.g. male/female, Yes/No
2. **Non-binary/polychotomous**, e.g. types of angina: Variant, stable, unstable.

Can be classified as:

1. Independent
2. Dependent

For example: Height depending on age. In this example, height is dependent variable, and age is independent variable.

Numeric data can also be classified as:

1. *Parametric:* A data set is said to be parametric if the values are normally distributed.
2. *Nonparametric*: A data set is said to be nonparametric if the values are not normally distributed.

These measures give us pattern or distribution of data series.

1. *Measures of central tendency:* Mean, median, mode
2. *Measures of dispersion:* Range, standard deviation, variance, quartiles

Statistics is broadly classified into 3 groups:

1. *Descriptive statistics:* Simply describe the data, e.g. frequency, counts, median, mean, graphs.
2. *Inferential statistics/hypothesis testing*: Comparison between different data sets.
3. *Statistical modelling*: It helps to make predictions from the study data set, e.g. logistic regression.

Data Distributions

1. **Normal distribution:** It is the most common and naturally occurring distribution of data. When the data set is represented graphically, a symmetric bell-shaped curve called Guassian curve is found.

Characteristics of Normal Distribution

1. Symmetric.
2. Bell shaped.

3. Mean, median, mode co-inside at a value of zero.
4. Single peaked, broad and flat tails on both sides.
5. One SD will include 68% of observations, 2SD—95.4%, 3SD—99.7%.

Skewness: When the data set is asymmetric, it is said to be positively or negatively skewed.

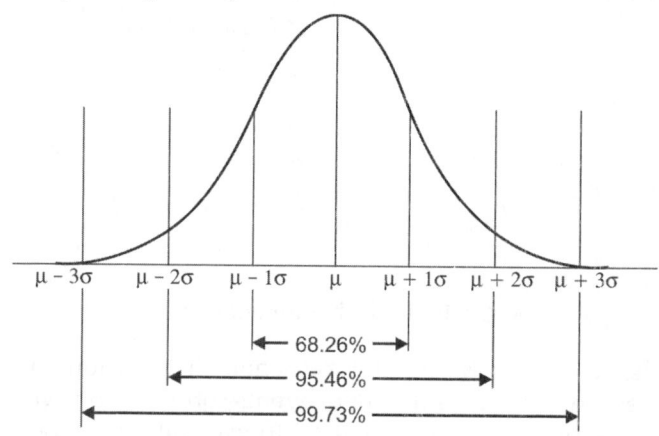

Fig. 20.1: Normal distribution of data (Gaussian curve)

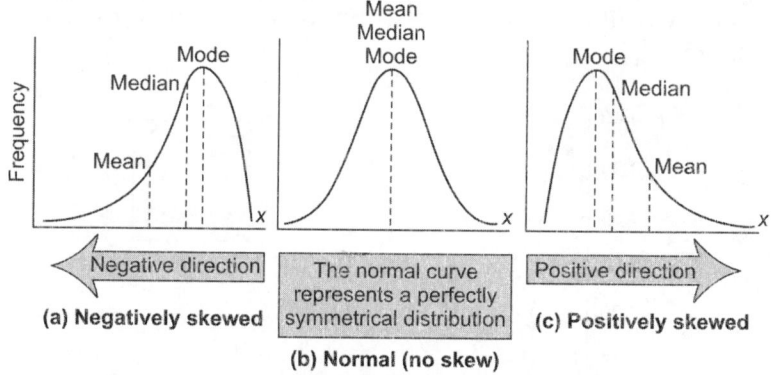

Fig. 20.2: Positive and negative skewness in the data

- *Negative skewed*: Tail towards the left. Mean<median< mode.
- *Positive skewed*: Long tail towards the right. Mean> median>mode.

Kurtosis: The property of peakness of the curve is called kurtosis. The value of kurtosis for a normal distribution curve is zero.

Bimodal/distribution of data: In this data distribution the graph has two distinct peaks, hence bimodal. For example, age distribution in Kaposi's sarcoma and Hodgkin's lymphoma.

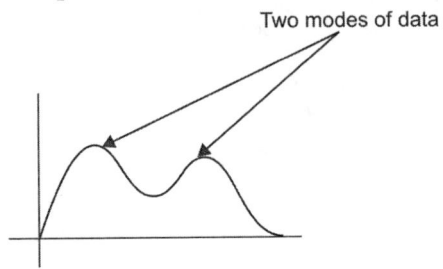

Fig. 20.3: Bimodal distribution of data

Poisson distribution: This type of data distribution is used to represent the data, i.e, number of events/observation occurring in specific time interval. It is used to calculate the probability of rare events in a continuous events of space or time. There is right-sided skewness in the graph when the mean is small. It resembles with the normal distribution curve when the mean is large.

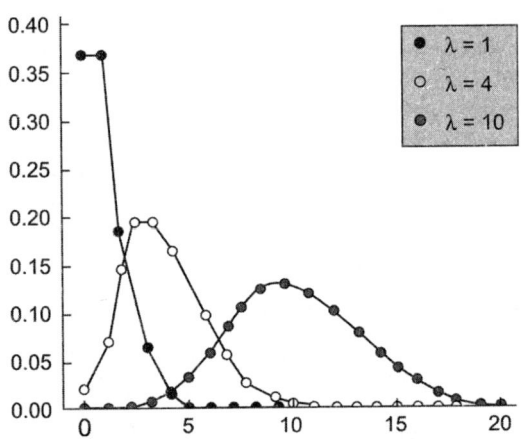

Fig. 20.4: Poisson distribution of data with changing means

Data Transformation

It is a mathematical manipulation done to each value to get a derived value, e.g. log transformation, reciprocals, square roots.

Uses of Log Transformation

1. Converts skewed distribution to normal distribution
2. To make an exponential curve to linear curve

For example, dose response curve

Z transformation: Deviation from the mean in units of SD.

These days requirement of data transformation has been reduced as different statistical softwares can deal with the actual values.

Measures of Central Tendency

1. **Mean:** It is the most common measure used in central tendency. There can be arithmetic mean and geometric mean:

   Arithmetic mean is the sum of all observations divided by the number of observations, e.g. haemoglobin values.

   Haemoglobin counts (Mean GM %) of anaemic females are as follows:
   - A: 9.5, B: 8.5, C: 7.9, D: 8.2, E: 9.2
   - Mean haemoglobin counts will be A + B + C + D + E/N (N = no. of observations)
   - It is denoted as sample mean—X and population mean as $\bar{X} = 8.66 \approx 8.7$

   Arithmetic mean is easily affected by extreme values. It is suitable for symmetric or normal distribution data. In case of skewed data, median is used.

   Geometric mean: It is calculated as nth root of product of n number of observations. It is used when the values are far apart, e.g. antibody titres, colony counts.

   Example: Total bilirubin count of a jaundice patient
   A—6, B—12
   GM = √6 × 12

2. **Median:** Median divides the data set into two equal halves. It is calculated after arranging the data in ascending or descending order. The central value is the median. In case

of odd number of measurements, the middle value is the median and in case of even number of measurements, the arithmetic mean of the 2 middle values gives the median.

Data set 1. Example: Height (in metre) of the girl student in class 10th.

A—1.54, B—1.48, C—1.61, D—1.51, E—1.60

Ascending order: B—1.48, D—1.51, **A—1.54**, C—1.61, E—1.60

Median: A—1.54

Data set 2. Example: Height (in metre) of the girl student in class 10th.

A—1.54, B—1.48, C—1.61, D—1.51

Ascending order: B—1.48, D—1.51, **A—1.54**, C—1.61

Median: $D + A/2 = 1.52$

Median is least affected by extreme values. It is used when the data is not normally distributed or skewed. The graph which is used to measure median is box and whisker plot.

3. **Mode:** The most frequently occurring value in the data series is the mode.

   Example: Weight of postmenopausal women in kg

   A—61, B—55, C—58, D—55

   Mode = 55

Graphical Representation of Data (Descriptive Statistics)

Descriptive statistics is simply describing the data in terms of count, frequency, average or graphs without comparison.

Graphical representation of data can be done by:

1. **Pie chart:** Used for categorical data. The sum of all percentages should be hundred (Fig. 20.5).
2. **Bar chart:** Used for quantitative data. They have 2 variants. They show mean and standard variation (Fig. 20.6).
   - *Multiple bar:* More than two values are compared simultaneously (Fig. 20.8).
   - *Stacked bar chart:* Two values are shown on the same bar; one over the other (Fig. 20.7).
3. **Histogram:** It gives the frequency distribution of the data set. (Fig. 20.9)
4. **Line diagram:** It depicts a trend in the data set with time.

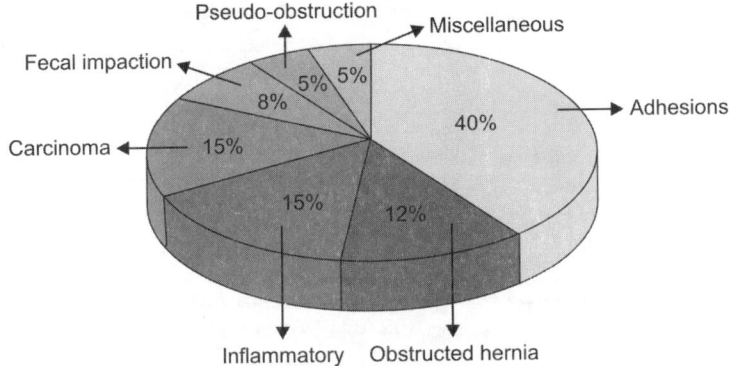

Fig. 20.5: Pie chart showing relative frequency of the underlying diagnosis of intestinal obstruction

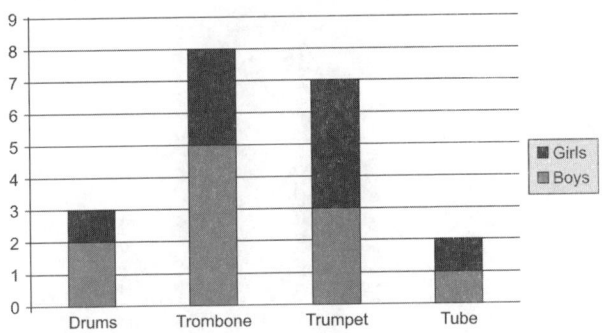

Fig. 20.6: Stacked bar chart

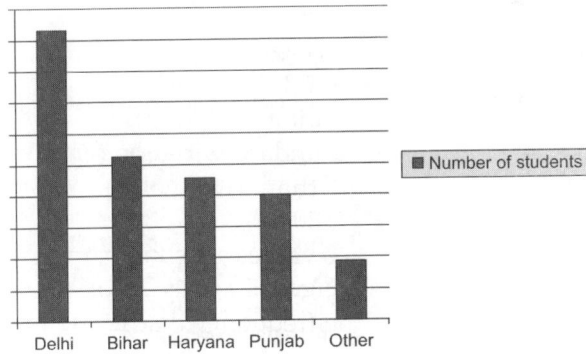

Fig. 20.7: Simple bar chart

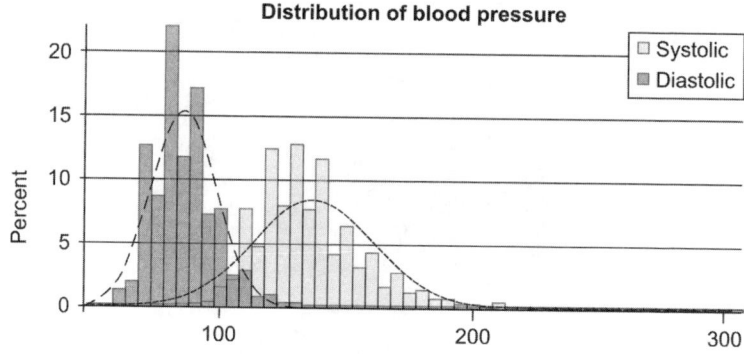

Fig. 20.8: Multiple bar chart

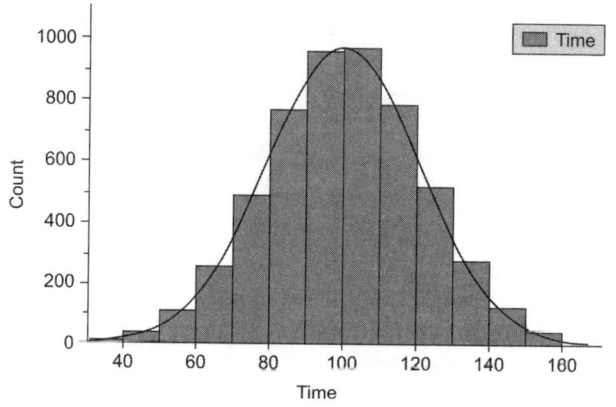

Fig. 20.9: Histogram

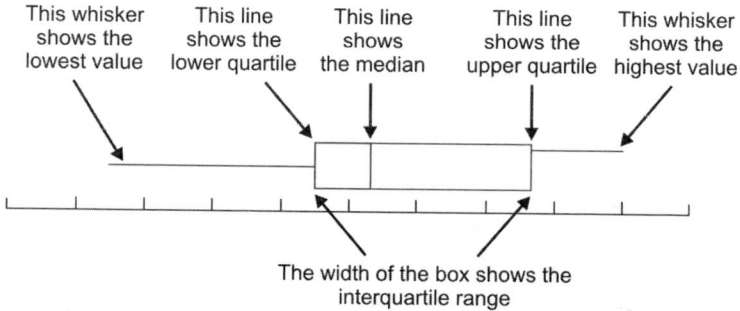

Fig. 20.10: Box and whisker plot

5. **Box and whiskers:** It is a five-figured summary of numerical data. It gives the range, median value, 25th and 75th percentile ends. This graph can be used to find extreme values, any value more than 1.5 times, the value of box are outliers (Fig. 20.10).

6. **Scatter plot:** Used to present association between two neumeric data sets. The dependent and independent variables are shown on x and y axis independently. For example, height vs weight. It can be extended to depict more than two variables by converting it into a bubble plot. The third variable is coded as radius of bubble, e.g. height vs weight vs body surface area (Fig. 20.11).

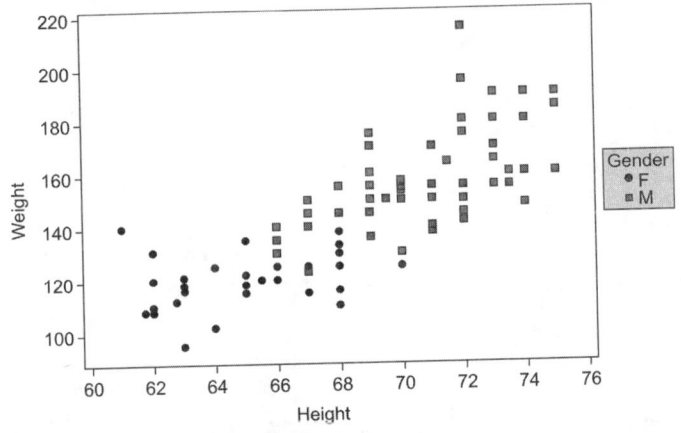

Fig. 20.11: Scatter plot of weight versus height

7. **Stem and leaf plot:** It can be used for small samples only. Weightage given to stem unit is 10 and leaf unit is one. It shows the actual value of each data on the plot.

8. **Kaplan-Meir plot/crazy staircase plot:** The depth and length of each staircase is not same. The X axis denotes time and Y axis denotes probability of survival. Used for survival analysis (Fig. 20.12).

9. **Forest plot:** It is the hallmark of meta-analysis as it summarises the results from different studies. The box represents odds ratio, size of box denotes sample size for individual study, the line extends up to 95% of CI and the diamond

denotes the summary or pooled result. Length of diamond depicts 95% CI. The vertical line passes through the odds ratio of 1. The forest plot is used in the logo of the Cochrane collaboration (Fig. 20.13).

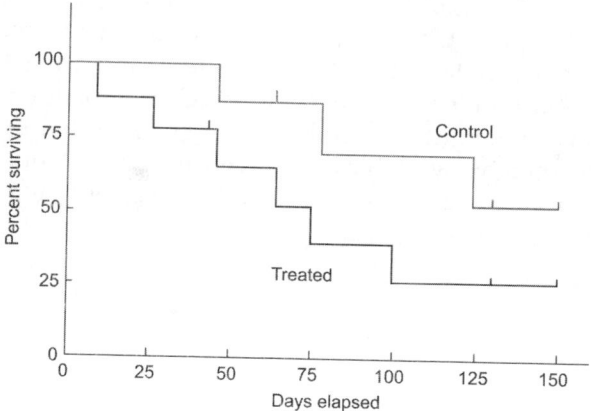

Fig. 20.12: Kaplan-Meir plot for survival analysis

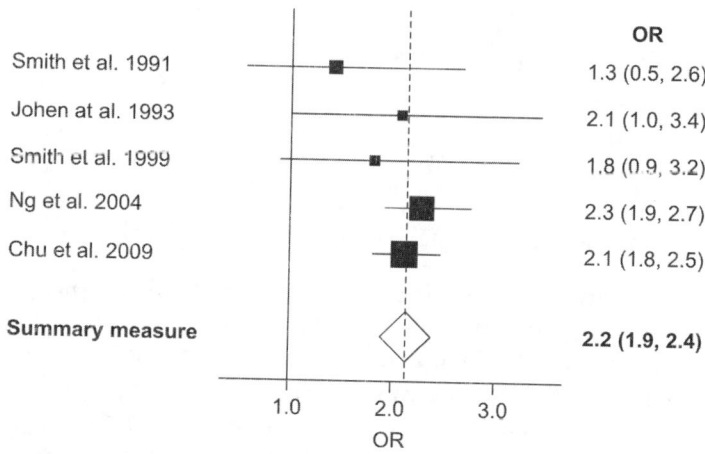

Fig. 20.13: Forest plot

Measures of Dispersion

1. **Range:** Difference between the highest and lowest value in a given data set, e.g. systolic blood pressure (mmHg) A–124, B–130, C–118, D–128

Range: 118–130

2. **Standard deviation:** This is also called root mean square deviation. It denotes how closely individual observations are located around the means, e.g. X_1—30, X_2—26, X_3—22

Mean ($\bar{X}$) = 26

$n = 3$

X	X–$\bar{X}$	(X–$\bar{X}$)²
30	4	16
26	0	0
22	–4	16
Sum		**32**

$$SD = \sqrt{\frac{\Sigma\left(X - \bar{X}\right)^2}{n - 1}}$$

SD = 4, Variance = 16

3. **Variance:** It is mean square deviation. It is calculated as square of standard deviation.

4. **Percentile and quartile:** Spread of data can be presented as ranking the values and then grouping them into hundred equal parts. Each group is called centile/percentile.

The median is represented as 50th percentile. Division of data into four equal part and each part is called quartile. The range of middle 50% of data is called inter-quartile range.

Example: You are the fourth tallest person in a group of 20. 80% of people are shorter than you.

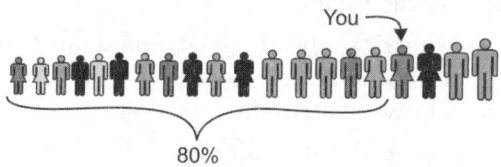

That means your are at the **80th percentile.**

If your height is 1.85 m, then '1.85 m' is the 80th percentile height in that group.

Hypothesis Testing

RESEARCH HYPOTHESIS

It is the research question/the main or primary objective of the study. Purpose is to analyze different data set and conclude if there is any statistically significant difference.

Hypothesis can be:

1. **Null hypothesis (H0):** It says that there is no difference between the two data sets. The difference observed is by chance (biological variability). This is the hypothesis which we hope for rejection in any research. The aim of the research is to prove the null hypothesis wrong.

2. **Alternative hypothesis (H1):** This says that there is a statistically significant difference between the two data set. For any research project the researcher hopes to prove the H1 to be true.

Steps in Hypothesis Testing

1. Research question should be framed and appropriate sample size should be calculated.

   From the following formula:

   $$N - 2(Z\alpha + Z\beta)^2 \times \sigma_1^2 + \sigma_2^2 / (\mu_1 - \mu_2)^2$$

   This is used to calculate the sample size for two group (mean) study.

   N—sample size, Zα—power index, Zα—0.05, Zβ—1.96, μ_1 and μ_2 means of the two groups, $\sigma_1 + \sigma_2$ standard deviation of two groups.

2. Finalise the statistical test to be applied for analysis of result and determine the p value by applying the test.
3. Compare the observed *p* value with the critical *p* value of 0.05–0.01 depending upon the study protocol.
4. If p value is more than the critical value, reject the null hypothesis.

p Value

It is the maximum probability of getting the observed difference by chance. If the *p* value is <0.05, the difference is said to be statistically significant. Lesser the *p* value, higher the statistical significance.

Errors While Testing the Hypothesis

There can be two types of errors
1. **Type 1(α):** False positive, actually there is no difference between the two data set but has found the difference. Incorrectly rejection of null hypothesis. It is more dangerous. It may lead to the introduction of the ineffective treatment option. The permissible value of alpha error is less than 0.05, i.e. 5%.Which means that 5 observations from 100 are false positive.
2. **Type 2(β):** False negative, actually there is difference between the two data set but the results fails to found the difference. Incorrectly accepting of null hypothesis.

It is less dangerous. The permissible value of beta error is less than 20%, i.e. 0.2.

Power of the Study

It is the probability of correctly rejecting null hypothesis when it is actually false.

Denoted as 1–β. That means minimum power required for the study is 1–β = 0.8.

There are 80% probability of correctly rejecting the null hypothesis.

Relation between the power and alpha error is reciprocal. These are the important determinants for sample size calculation.

		Truth about the population	
		H_o true	H_a true
Decision based on sample	Reject H_o	Type I error	Correct decision
	Accept H_a	Correct decision	Type II error

P-value

It is the maximum probability of getting the observed result by chance. It is predefined in the protocol before the initiation of the protocol. It is considered statistically significant if the p value is < 0.05. Further lesser the value more will be the credibility of the study. It is important to have an adequate sample size to have a true value. With larger the sample size, chances of getting a significant difference is higher than with the smaller sample. Highly significant p value is not indicative of clinical application of the result. Hence to make it more valuable, it is given with related confidence interval (CI).

Confidence interval: It is defined as the range calculated from the study sample that is expected to contain the true population value.

Confidence level: Probability that the interval actual contents the true values.

Formula for calculation of CI means

$$\text{CI Means} = \text{Mean} \pm Z \times \text{SEM}$$

Example: Student calculated haemoglobin levels in 100 patients and found the mean to be 12.5 ± SD 3.6. So CI (95%) will be calculated as:

$$= 12.5\ (\pm 1.96) \times 3.6/\sqrt{100} = \text{CI}\ (3.79 - 5.21)$$

Hence from the above formula lesser is the confidence interval more accurate is the result. This is achieved by increasing the sample size.

Statistical Tests

Depending on the type of research question and the data to be analysed specific type of statistical tests need to be applied. Initially this analysis was done manually using mathematical formulae but with the availability of different statistical softwares (statistical package for social sciences—spss, statistical analysis software—sas, graphpad prism), meagre knowledge of a few tests is enough to analyze different data sets. These tests are usually named after the scientists who introduced them followed by the statistical parameters whose value we obtain after applying the test.

To test normality of data distribution
- Kolmogorov-Smirnov test
- Shapiro-Wilk test

To Compare Difference between Unpaired/Independent Data Sets

For Numeric Data

- **Parametric:** Two groups—unpaired students t test, >2 groups—ANOVA
- **Non-parametric:** Two groups—Mann-Whitney U test, >2 groups—Kruskall-Wallis test

For Categorical Data

- 2 groups—Chi square (χ^2) test, Fisher's exact test, >2 groups—chi-square test

To Compare Difference between Paired/Dependent Data Sets

For Numeric Data

- *Parametric:* 2 groups—paired students t test, >2 groups— Repeated measures ANOVA
- *Non-parametric:* 2 groups—Wilcoxons matched pairs signed rank test, >2 groups—Friedman's ANOVA

For Categorical Data

- 2 groups—McNemar's test, >2 groups—Cochran's Q test

To Establish if there is any Correlation between Groups

For Numeric Data

- *Parametric:* Pearsons r
- *Non-parametric:* Spearman's p, Kendall's *t* test

For Categorical Data

- *2*2 data*: Relative risk, odds ratio
- *Others:* Chi-square for trends, logistic regression

To Compare Survival Plots or Other Time Trend (Cancer Studies)

- Log rank test
- Cox-Mantel test

To Establish Agreement for Diagnostic, Screening or Rating Assessment

For Numeric Data

- Intra-class correlation coefficient

For Categorical Data

- Cohen's kappa statistic

DIAGNOSTIC TESTS

Application

These tests are used to evaluate diagnostic and screening method before adopting them in clinical practice.

Even clinical examination procedures and scoring system are examples of such diagnostic test:

The truth

Test score:	Has the disease	Does not have the disease	
Positive	True positives (TP)	False positives (TP)	$PPV = \dfrac{TP}{TP + FP}$
Negative	True negatives (TP)	False negatives (TP)	$NPV = \dfrac{TP}{TP + FN}$

Sensitivity	Specificity
$\dfrac{TP}{TP + FN}$	$\dfrac{TP}{TP + FP}$

Or, $\dfrac{a}{a + c}$ $\dfrac{d}{d + b}$

Fig. 22.1

1. **Sensitivity:** Probability of getting a positive result when patient has the disease
2. **Specificity:** Probability of getting a negative result when patient does not have the disease
3. **Positive predictive value:** The probability of subject being diseased when the test is positive
4. **Negative predictive value:** The probability of subject being healthy when the test is negative.
5. **Likelihood ratios:** It is used by the clinician to predict the risk of disease in patient if prior probability of disease is known by using sensitivity and specificity.
   Likelihood ratio of a positive test result (lr+) = sensitivity / 1– specificity
   Likelihood ratio of a negative test result (lr-) = 1– Sensitivity / specificity

Minor Details of Statistical Test

Student t-Test

This test is used to compare numeric/quantitative data between two groups. This test is introduced by statistician William Sealy Gosset.

It can be of two types depending upon the variable to be compared, i.e. dependent or independent.

TABLE 22.1: Selecting statistical tests

Measurement scale of the dependent variable	One independent variable				Two independent variables	
	Two levels		More than 2 levels		Factorial designs	
	Two independent groups	Two dependent groups	Multiple independent groups	Multiple dependent groups	Independent groups	Dependent groups
Interval or ratio	Independent t-test	Dependent t-test	One-way ANOVA	Repeated measures ANOVA	Two-factor ANOVA	Two-factor ANOVA repeated measures
Ordinal	Mann-Whitney U	Wilcoxon	Kruskal-Walls	Friedman		
Nominal	Chi-square		Chi-square		Chi-square	

Paired Student t-Test—Dependent Variable

Comparison of the same parameter before and after giving drug.

Unpaired Student t-Test—Independent

Comparison of the variables in control and test group.

Pre-requisite: Minimum sample size has to be 30. Theoretically it can be applied to the less sample size as much as 10. But the data has to be normally distributed.

Student's *t*-distribution

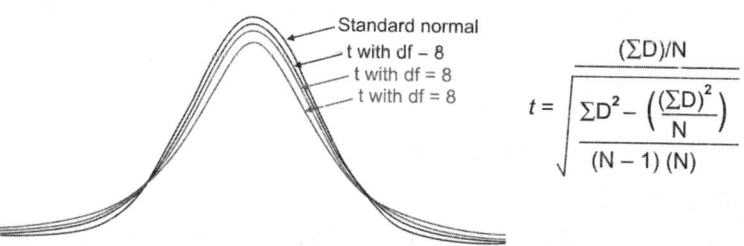

$$t = \sqrt{\dfrac{(\Sigma D)/N}{\dfrac{\Sigma D^2 - \left(\dfrac{(\Sigma D)^2}{N}\right)}{(N-1)(N)}}}$$

Fig. 22.2: 't' distribution formula for '*t*' score

It depends upon *t* distribution curve: This is little broader and flatter than the normal distribution curve (as shown in the graph).

Normally test is two-tailed evaluation. In some cases it can be one-tailed also, e.g. studying the effect of drug on height.

D-Sum of the Differences

In this formula the sum of the differences between means is the numerator. Denominator is the variance within the samples.

ANOVA (ANALYSIS OF VARIANCE)

It is used to compare numeric data in two or more groups. This is applicable when data is normally distributed. It is a misnomer where it compares the means rather than variance. The ratio of two variances is compared to decide whether the means are different or not. One-way ANOVA is used to compare the means of single independent variables. Multifactor ANOVA is used to compare means of different independent variables. The distribution curve is called "F" distribution curve.

Example: Comparison of three treatment groups for hypertension.

	Group A (B- blockers)	Group B (CCBs)	Group C(Diuretics)
Effect on BP			

After applying ANOVA post-HOC test is applied.

MANOVA (MULTIPLE ANALYSIS OF VARIANCE)

This test is used when there are two or more dependent variables, e.g. in the above study to compare the different treatment hypertension with or without salt restriction.

Chi-Square Test

This test was introduced by Karl Pearson. This test compares categorical data (percentages or proportions) in two or more groups, e.g. gender, marital status. This is applicable to the sample size ≥ 50. This is denoted as χ^2. It is calculated by using contingency table. It is calculated as $-\sum(O - E)^2/E$,

O—observed frequency and E—expected frequency. A low value of chi-square means there is a high co-relation between your two sets of data. The p value is found out from chi-square distribution. Fisher's exact test can also be used to compare the percentages or proportions from two groups. There are different types of chi-square tests.

1. **Chi-square test for trends:** Assess the significant trends in the incidence of disease, e.g. incidence of diabetes with respect to age, socioeconomic status.
2. **Chi-square goodness of fit:** Compare the observed frequency with the standard.
3. **McNemar chi-square test:** Use to compare the groups in a paired situation.

Chi-Square Distribution

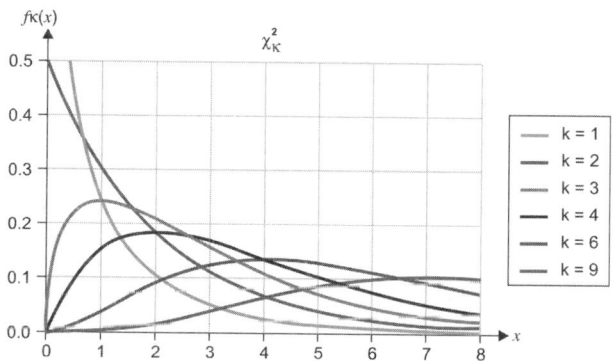

Fig. 22.3: Chi-square distribution. IT is right-sided skewed curve. As the degree of freedom (sample size–1), it becomes normally distributed

Example: Smoking profile

	Present	Absent	Row total
Group 1	A	B	A+B
Group 2	C	D	C+D
Column total	A+C	B+D	A+B+C+D

$$p = (A + B) \times (C + D) \times (A + C) \times (B + D)/(ABCD)(A + B + C + D)$$

BIBLIOGRAPHY

1. Mahendra N Parikh et al, Research Methodology simplified every clinician a researcher, New Delhi, Jaypee Brothers, 1st edition, 2010.

Section D

Special Topics

- ➲ Paediatric Pharmacology
- ➲ Geriatric Pharmacology
- ➲ Drug Use in Pregnancy
- ➲ New Drug Delivery System
- ➲ Chronopharmacology
- ➲ Drug Transporters
- ➲ Ion Channels
- ➲ Phosphodiesterase (PDE) Inhibitors
- ➲ Stem Cell Therapy

Paediatric Pharmacology

Paediatric population are not the small adult, they differ in various pharmacokinetics and pharmacodynamics from adults. Adults and children respond to drugs differently. Paediatrics drug should be administered in suitable formulation, dosage and route of administration. Medications that are used commonly in paediatric practice do have well-articulated details such as age/weight dosing, implications for breast-feeding and important information related to drug absorption, distribution, elimination and adverse events. All pharmacokinetic parameters are change as age and dosage should be adjusted accordingly.

TABLE 23.1: Age group of paediatric population

Term	Age
Preterm/premature	<36 weeks gestation
Neonate	<30 days
Infant	1 month to 1 year
Child	1–12 years
Adoloscent	12–18 years

PAEDIATRIC DOSAGE FORMS

- **Elixirs:** Alcoholic solution. Drug molecules dissolved. No need of shaking
- **Suspensions:** Insoluble substances dissolved in uniformly in a solvent. Risk of administering unequal doses if not shaken well. High dose can lead to toxicity, caution to mother.

- **Drops:** Convenient and precise dosing
- **Powders:** Easy to mix with food and drink. Provide large surface area for absorption.

Compliance

Difficult to achieve because	How to improve it
1. Inability to follow directions	Pill boxes
	Complete the full course of treatment
2. Measuring errors	Calibrated medicine spoons/syringes
3. Spilling and spitting out	Repeat the dose

Dose Calculation

- Dose calculated as mg/kg
- Various parameters used to calculate dose are age, weight and surface area.
- Based on age:

  Child dose = age/age + 12 × adult dose   (Young's formula)

  Child dose = age/20 × adult dose   (Dilling's formula)
- Based on weight

  Paediatric dose = body weight/70 x average adult dose
- Based on body surface area = (BSA)

  Paediatric dose = BSA/1.7 × average adult dose

  Body surface area (BSA) provides a more accurate basis for dose calculation, because total body water, extracellular fluid volume and metabolic activity are better paralleled by BSA.

  The BSA of an individual can be calculated from Dubois formula:

  $$BSA\ (m^2) = BW\ (kg)\ 0.425 \times Height\ (cm)\ 0.725 \times 0.007184$$

  It can also be obtained from chart-form or slide-rule nomograms which is based on BW and height.

PHYSIOLOGICAL DIFFERENCES IN PAEDIATRIC POPULATION

Table 23.2 gives a summary of pharmacokinetic parameters compared to that of adult.

TABLE 23.2: Pharmacokinetic parameters

Parameters	Neonate (<1 month) Infant (1 month to 1 year)	Adoles-cent	Clinical relevance
Absorption			
Drug absorption			• *Increased*: Penicillins • *Decreased*: Paracetomol, phenobarbitone, phenytoin
Gastric acidity	Decreased	Normal	• Drugs with an acidic pH Reduce and unpredictable absorption, e.g. penicillin. • Normal adult gastric acid secretions are achieved by about 3 years of age.
GI motility	Decreased	Normal	• During infancy the absorption of drugs that are absorbed in the stomach is increased • However, drugs absorbed from the intestine will have a decreased or possibly delayed absorption
Blood flow to absorbing area	Unpredicatble	Normal	• Absorption of certain drugs like digoxine, aminogly-cosides and anticonvulsants may be variable
Skin permeability	Increased	Normal	• Topical/injections • Transdermal absorption faster
Rectal absorption	Increased	Normal	• Preferred route for diazepam administration for febrile convulsion
Concen-tration of bile acid and lipase	Low	Normal	• Decrease absorption of lipid soluble drugs, e.g. phenobarbitone
Blood–brain barrier permeability	Increased	Normal	• Physiological jaundice • Unconjugated bilirubin crosses BBB—kernicterus • Sulphonamide— kernicterus • Displacement of bilirubin from PPB

Contd.

Parameters	Neonate (<1 month) Infant (1 month to 1 year)	Adolescent	Clinical relevance
Plasma proteins	Significantly decreased	Normal	• Free concentration of drug with high PPB will be very high, e.g. NSAIDs, anticonvulsants, sulphonamide, warfarin. • Dose will be reduced • Phenytoin: Therapeutic range for neonates = 6–15 mg/kg • Therapeutic range for children and adults = 10–20 mg/kg
Total body water and extracellular fluid volume thus	Increased		• Larger doses of water-soluble drugs are required, e.g. aminoglycosides, digoxin
Liver enzymes	Immature till 1st year of the life. After 1st year, liver enzymes may be raised	Normal	• Decreased enzyme for glucuronidation: Chloramphenicol toxicity: Gray baby syndrome • Paracetamol toxicity in neonates • Increased metabolism: Theophylline, phenytoin, carbamazepine
GFR	Decreased At birth- 30–40% of adult 3rd week – 50–60% Adult value By 1st year – Normal	Normal	• Aminoglycosides—t1/2 Increased • Penicillins and cephalosporins have long duration, hence dosage and frequency should be reduced. • Ampicillin • At birth—50–100 mg/kg/day to be divided in two doses

Contd.

Parameters	Neonate (<1 month) Infant (1 month to 1 year)	Adoles-cent	Clinical relevance
			• After 1 week—100–200 mg/kg/day to be divided in three doses
Renal blood flow	Decreased	Normal	
Tubular secretion	Decreased	Normal	• Penicillins, cephalosporin—t1/2 increased • Clearance is 34% of adult value
Receptor sensitivity	Increased		• Neonates and infants are more susceptible for CNS depressant drugs, e.g. opioids—reduce functioning Pgp (efflux transporter) at BBB • Indomethacin administration causes rapid closure of PDA 　• COX is more sensitive to NSAID inhibition
Adverse drug reactions	Increased		• Neonate and children are susceptible to special ADR • Growth suppression with steroids • Discolouration of teeth-tetracyclines • closure of epiphysis/stunting—androgens • Rey's syndrome—aspirin in viral fever • Metoclopramide induced—acute muscular dystonia

BIBLIOGRAPHY

1. Katzung DG, Basic and Clinical Pharmacology, Chapter 59, Special Aspect of Perinatal and Paediatric Pharmacology, New York, McGraw-Hill Education Publishing, 2018 (14th edition).

Geriatric Pharmacology

Society has traditionally classified everyone over 65 as "elderly", but most authorities consider the field of geriatrics to apply to persons over 75 even though this too is an arbitrary definition.

Why elders need special precaution while prescribing:
1. Age related changes.
2. Altered pharmacokinetic and pharmacodynamics of drug
3. Suffering from multiple diseases and symptoms
4. Higher rates of polypharmacy
5. Incidence of adverse drug reactions are more common
6. Noncompliance with treatment

PHYSIOLOGICAL CHANGES

Steady decline in functional capacities of major organ systems begins around the age of 45 years.

Age related changes in elderly affecting the pharmacokinetic and pharmacodynamics of drug.

PHARMACOKINETIC AND DYNAMIC CHANGES

Absorption

- Certain factors like reduced gastric acid secretion, altered nutritional habits, greater consumption of nonprescription drugs like antacids and laxative will cause increase gastric pH and impairment in the absorption of iron and calcium.
- Delayed gastric emptying, decreased total surface area of absorption, reduced GI blood flow may cause delayed onset

TABLE 24.1: Physiological changes with age

Physiological parameter	Change	Application
Body water	Reduced	Vd will be reduced Digoxin (high Vd)—loading dose is reduced
Lean body mass	Reduced	Vd will be reduced
Serum albumin	Reduced	Weak acidic drugs like aspirin, barbiturates—free concentration increased.
Renal clearance	Reduced	Aminoglycoside T1/2—increased Dose and frequency—reduced Maintenance dose of digoxin—reduced
Hepatic blood flow	Reduced	Reduced hepatic metabolism of the drug. High bioavailability of the drug with high hepatic extraction—lignocaine. Higher chances of toxicity with propranolol.

of action and/or lower serum levels of drugs necessitating dose adjustment.

Distribution

- 20 to 30% reduction in total body water content, increased in serum levels of water soluble drugs such as lithium with increased risk of side effects.
- 25 30% increase in body fat, prolongs half-life of lipid soluble drugs acting on CNS, e.g. psychotropics (benzodiazepine, phenobarbitone, opioids)—increased risk of side effects.
- Reduced plasma proteins leading to higher free plasma concentration of high protein bound drugs like NASIDs, sulfonylurea, warfarin. This requires dose adjustment.

Metabolism

- Decreased liver cell mass and 35% decreased liver blood flow, an important variable in the clearance of drugs that have a high hepatic extraction ratio.
- The greatest changes are in phase I reactions, decreased activity of CYP—450 enzymes—increased risk of adverse drug–drug interactions.
- Decreased phase I reactions—oxidation, reduction, hydroxylation—decreased metabolism—needing dose adjustment.

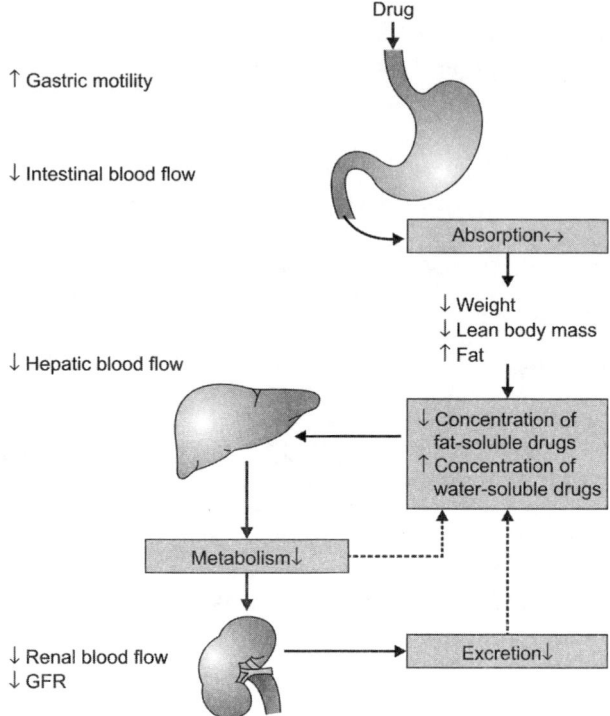

Fig. 24.1: Physiological changes with age

- There are much smaller changes in the ability of the liver to carry out conjugation (phase II) reactions.

Significant Effect of Age on Hepatic Clearance of Drugs

Benzodiazepine: Diazepam, flurazepam, alprazolam, clobazam, chlordiazepoxide, **NSAIDs:** Phenylbutazone, **OHA:** Tolbutamide, **TCAs:** Imipramine, meperidine, nortriptyline, **B-blocker:** Propranolol, drugs like quinidine, quinine, theophylline.

Drug Elimination

Age related changes in renal function are as follows:
1. Loss of glomeruli.
2. Decrease renal blood flow,
3. Fall in GFR and tubular function: 1% fall in GFR/year from age > 40, renal excreted drug needs dose adjustment.

The practical result of this change is marked prolongation of the half-life of many drugs. An adjustment in dose and frequency of drug use is required.

Serum creatinine is not a good indicator of renal function test as there is a reduction in lean body mass with age.

For more precise calculations Cockcroft and Gault formula is used. The formula is as follows:

Creatinine clearence (mg/ml) =

$$(140 - age) (wt.\ in\ kg)/72^* \text{ serum creatinine}$$

For females multiplication factor is 0.85.

The lungs are important for the excretion of volatile drugs. As a result of reduced respiratory capacity and the increased incidence of active pulmonary disease in the elderly, the use of inhalation anaesthesia is less common and parenteral agents more common in this age group.

Pharmacodynamic Changes

Elderly may respond differently to a given dose of drugs as compared to younger. They are more "sensitive" to the action of many drugs. Generally lower doses are required to achieve the same effect with advancing age

Increased sensitivity is due to:

1. Change in receptors sensitivity and postreceptors alterations, e.g. decrease in responsiveness to β-adrenoceptor agonists, sensitivity to the sedative hypnotics and analgesics is increased.
2. **Blunting homeostatic responses:** Increase incidence of symptomatic orthostatic hypotension.

    The average 2-hour postprandial blood glucose level increases by about 1 mg/dL for each year of age above 50. Glycemic control may be difficult to achieve.
3. Temperature regulation is also impaired, and hypothermia is poorly tolerated by the elderly.

SUFFERING FROM MULTIPLE DISEASES AND SYMPTOMS

Most common problems seen in elderly people are:

Disease related: Incontinence, infection, immunodeficiency, impaired vision and auditory sense, impaction of faeces, hypertension, diabetes mellitus, arthritis, ischemic heart disease, Alzheimer's disease.

Psychological problems: Immobility, isolation, intellectual loss, depression insomnia, dementia.

INCIDENCE OF ADVERSE DRUG REACTIONS ARE MORE COMMON

Incidence of ADR is 2 to 3 times that found in young adults. Following are the examples:

1. **Postural hypotension:** Isosornidedinitrate, TCAs, antipsychotics, leveodopa.
2. **Constipation:** Anticholinergics, antidepressants, antipsychotics, opioids, nifedipine.
3. **Urinary incontinence:** B-blockers, diuretics.
4. **Parkinsonism:** Antipsychotic, metochlopramice.
5. **Depression:** Sedative, anxiolytics.
6. **Confusional state:** Anticholinergics, anticonvulsants, theophyllins.
7. **Vitamin deficiencies:** Alcohol—vitamin B_1 and B_{12}, antacid—reduced absorption of iron, hypophosphotemia, phenytoin—vitamin K, megaloblasticanaemia
8. **Anticholinergics:** Urinary retention and glaucoma.

HIGHER RATES OF POLYPHARMACY

- Multiple concomitant disorder and multiple drugs for that— can cause drug interactions and ADR.

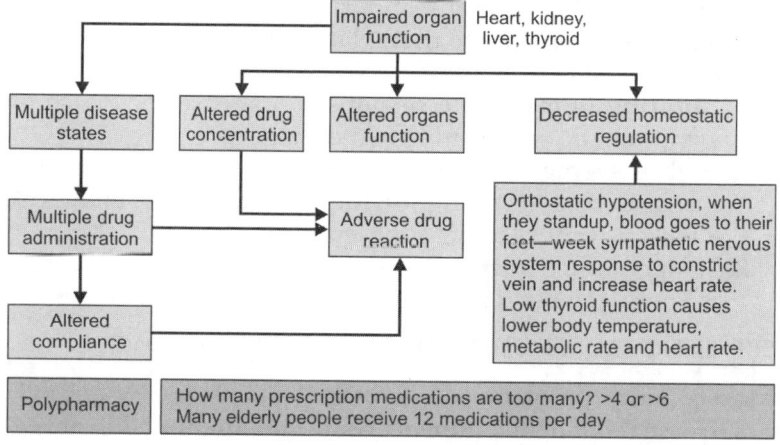

Fig. 24.2: Factors contributing to adverse drug reaction in elderly patients

- Negligence as a process of aging, e.g. hearing loss, etc
- They have a tendency to change the doctor.

NON-COMPLIANCE

Reasons why elderly have compliance problems for taking medications:

- Difficulty in opening pill containers (weak/arthritis pain/tremors/spills).
- Difficulty in reading the labels and information.
- *Depression:* Can lead to sleepy and poor concept of time for doses.
- *Cognitive impairment:* Cannot recall a few moments ago.
- *Cost of medications are prohibitive:* Food vs. medications (lack of economical security).
  Various ways to improve noncompliance:
  - Patient education, psychological and moral support.
  - Use of medicine calendars/records.
  - Simplifying drug regimens.
  - Link it with meals.
  - Use of similar schedules.
  - Easy handling and opening of bottles.
  - Large labels with boldly written instructions on containers and package inserts.

Practical Aspects of Geriatric Pharmacology

A few principles of geriatric pharmacology:

1. Take a careful drug history.
2. Prescribe only for a specific and rational indication.
3. Define the goal of drug therapy.
4. Maintain a high index of suspicion regarding drug reactions and interactions. Know what other drugs the patient is taking, including over-the-counter.
5. Simplify the regimen as much as possible.

BIBLIOGRAPHY

1. Katzung DG, Basic and Clinical Pharmacology, Chapter 59, Special aspect of perinatal and paediatric pharmacology, New York, McGraw-Hill Education Publishing, 2018 (14th edition).

Drug Use in Pregnancy

Prescribing for the pregnant woman requires a lot of skill and restraint.

- There is potential for harmful effects on the growing foetus.
- Maternal medication can also increase the incidence of abortion, foetal death, premature/delayed labour or create perinatal problems.
- Because of human variation, subtle effects to the foetus may be virtually impossible to identify.
- There are pronounced and progressive physiological changes during pregnancy which can affect drug disposition.
- There is notable paucity of and difficulties in research in this area.
- Assume all drugs are harmful until proven otherwise.

Pharmacokinetic Changes seen in Pregnancy

Critical factors affecting placental drug transfer and drug effects on the fetus include the following:

1. **The physiological properties of the drug:** Drug passage across the placenta is dependent on lipid solubility and degree of drug ionization. Lipophilic drugs tend to diffuse readily across the placenta and enter the foetal circulation, e.g. thiopental, a drug commonly used for cesarean sections, crosses the placenta almost immediately and can produce sedation or apnea in the newborn infant. Highly ionized drugs such as succinylcholine and tubocurarine, also used for caesarean sections, cross the placenta

slowly and achieve very low concentrations in the foetus. Impermeability of the placenta to polar compounds is relative rather than absolute. If high enough maternal-foetal concentration gradients are achieved, polar compounds cross the placenta in measurable amounts.

2. **Molecular size and pH:** The molecular weight of the drug also influences the rate of transfer and the amount of drug transferred across the placenta, depending upon their lipid solubility and degree of ionization. An important clinical application of this property is the choice of heparin as an anticoagulant in pregnant women. Because it is a very large (and polar) molecule, heparin is unable to cross the placenta. Unlike warfarin, which is teratogenic and should be avoided during the first trimester and even beyond (as the brain continues to develop), heparin may be safely given to pregnant women who need anticoagulation.

3. **Placental transporters:** Several drug transporters of the ABC (ATP binding cassette) and SLC (solute carrier) families are present in the placenta, such as P-glycoprotein, breast cancer resistance protein, or organic anion/cation transporters. Hence the passage of drugs across the placenta can no longer be predicted simply on the basis of their physical-chemical properties. P-glycoprotein encoded by the MDR1 gene pumps back into the maternal circulation a variety of drugs, e.g. vinblastine, doxorubicin. Viral protease inhibitors, which are substrates of P-glycoprotein, achieve only low foetal concentrations an effect that may increase the risk of vertical HIV infection from the mother to the foetus. The hypoglycemic drug glyburide shows much lower concentrations in the foetus as compared to the mother as it is effluxed from the foetal circulation by the BCRP and MRP3 transporters.

4. **Protein binding:** The degree to which a drug is bound to plasma proteins may also affect the rate and extent of transfer, e.g. sulfonamides, barbiturates, phenytoin, glyburide and local anaesthetic agents. Very high maternal protein binding contributes to lower foetal levels as compared to maternal concentrations.

5. **Placental and foetal drug metabolism:** The placenta expresses a variety of xenobiotic-metabolizing enzymes

from the earlier stages of pregnancy. However, compared to the liver, placental drug metabolism seems to be relatively minor and does not significantly limit the extent of drug delivery to the foetus. On the other hand, placental enzymes can catalyze the formation of reactive metabolites that might be fetotoxic. Drugs which have been shown to undergo significant placental metabolism include azidothymidine, dexamethasone, and prednisolone. The anticonvulsant oxcarbazepine is also metabolized to some extent by the human placenta.

Altered Physiology in Pregnancy

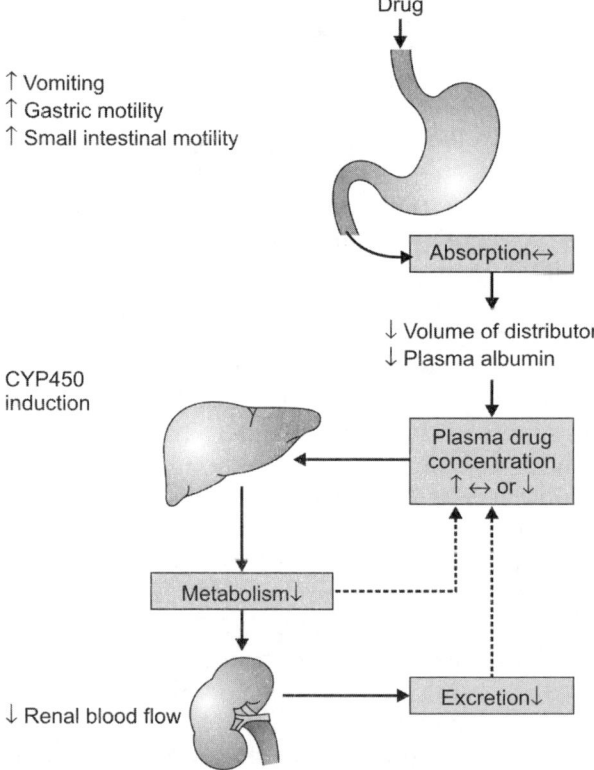

Fig. 25.1: Physiological changes in pregnancy

Absorption

- Gastric emptying and small intestinal motility are reduced.
- Vomiting associated with pregnancy may make oral drug administration impractical.

Distribution

- Blood volume increases by one-third, with expansion in plasma volume.
- Reduced hematocrit value.
- Increase in body water due to a larger extravascular volume. Its clinical significance is increased volume of distribution. For water-soluble drugs, although clearance is unaltered, their half-life is prolonged.
- During pregnancy, the plasma protein concentration falls. However, the concentration of free drug usually remains unaltered, because a greater volume of distribution of free drug is accompanied by increased clearance of free drug.

Metabolism

- Metabolism of drugs by the liver is increased, largely due to enzyme induction but blood flow remains unchanged.
- Rate of elimination of those drugs (e.g. theophylline), for which enzyme activity rather than liver blood flow is the main determinant of elimination rate is increased.

Renal Excretion

- Excretion of drugs via the kidney increases
- Renal plasma flow almost doubles
- Glomerular filtration rate increases by two-thirds during pregnancy

Potential harmful effects on the growing foetus depends upon the

1. Rate at which the drug crosses the placenta and the amount of drug reaching the foetus;
2. Duration of exposure to the drug
3. Distribution characteristics in different foetal tissues
4. Stage of placental and foetal development at the time of exposure to the drug; and
5. Effects of drugs used in combination

Principles of prescribing in pregnancy
- Where possible use nondrug therapy.
- Prescribe drugs only when definitely needed.
- Choose the drug having the best safety record over time.
- Avoid newer drugs, unless safety is clearly established.
- Over-the-counter drugs cannot be assumed to be safe.
- As far as possible avoid medication in first 10 weeks of pregnancy.
- Use the lowest effective dose.
- Use drugs for the shortest period necessary.
- If possible, give drug intermittently.

PHARMACODYNAMICS

A. Maternal Drug Actions

Drug effects on other maternal tissues are not changed significantly by pregnancy, although the physiological parameters like cardiac output, renal blood flow, etc. may be altered, requiring the use of drugs that are not needed by the same woman when she is not pregnant.

For example, cardiac glycosides and diuretics may be needed for heart failure precipitated by the increased cardiac workload of pregnancy, or insulin may be required for control of blood glucose in pregnancy-induced diabetes.

B. Therapeutic Drug Actions in the Foetus

This involves drug administration to the pregnant woman with the foetus as the target of the drug. Several issues, including ethical and legal considerations, are particular to foetal medicine, e.g. corticosteroids are used to stimulate foetal lung maturation when preterm birth is expected.

    a. Phenobarbital, when given to pregnant women near term, can induce foetal hepatic enzymes responsible for the glucuronidation of bilirubin, and the incidence of jaundice is lower in newborns.

    b. Antiarrhythmic drugs have also been given to mothers for treatment of foetal cardiac arrhythmias. Although their efficacy has not yet been established by controlled studies, digoxin, flecainide, procainamide, verapamil, and other antiarrhythmic agents have been shown to be effective in case series.

c. Maternal use of zidovudine decreases by two-thirds transmission of HIV from the mother to the foetus, and use of combinations of three antiretroviral agents can eliminate foetal infection almost entirely.

C. Teratogenic Drug Actions

A single intrauterine exposure to a drug can affect the foetal structures undergoing rapid development at the time of exposure.

TABLE 25.1: Examples of drugs having teratogenic effects

Drug	Adverse effect
Thalidomide	Phocomelia (seal limbs), multiple defects
Tetracycline	Discoloured and deformed teeth, retarded bone growth
Phenytoin	Hypoplastic phalanges, cleft lip/palate, microcephaly
Valproate	Spina bifida and neural tube defect
Warfarin	Depressed nose; eye and hand defects, growth retardation
Alcohol	Low IQ baby, growth retardation, foetal alcohol syndrome
Estrogen	Vaginal adenocarcinoma in female offspring
ACE inhibitors	Hypoplasia of organs, growth retardation, foetal loss
Indomethacin/aspirin	Premature closure of ductus arteriosus
Antithyroid drugs	Foetal goitre and hypothyroidism
Lithium	Foetal goitre, cardiac and other abnormalities
Isotretinoin	Craniofacial, heart and CNS defects

TABLE 25.2: US-FDA classification for risk category of drug use in pregnancy

Category	Criteria	Drug
A	Safety proven	Inj. Mag. sulfate, thyroxine
B	Inadequate data available Use—Benefit > Risk	Penicillins, erythromycin, paracetamol
C	Inadequate data available Use—Benefit > Risk	Morphine codeine corticosteroid, atropine

Contd.

TABLE 25.2: US-FDA classification for risk category of drug use in pregnancy (*Contd.*)

Category	Criteria	Drug
D	Teratogenic potential Risk vs benefit ratio goes in favour of their use	Aspirin, anticonvulsant
X	Absolutely contraindicated outweighs possible benefit	Isotretinoin, estrogen, methotrexate, ACE inhibitors, ARB

TABLE 25.3: Effect of drug on foetal growth depending on foetal age

Days	Period	Teratogenic effect	
17 days	Fertilization and implantation	Loss of pregnancy	Methotrexate: Rheumatoid arthritis
18 to 55 days	Organogenesis	Deformities are produced	Phenytoin—foetal hydantoin
56 days onwards	Growth and development	Developmental and functional abnormalities	ACE inhibitors: Hypoplasia of organs, lungs and kidneys NSAIDs: Premature closure of ductus arteriosus.

DRUG USE IN LACTATION

Principle of prescribing in lactation: Administration of drug in a lactating mother may affect breast milk secretion or may affect baby adversely through milk. pH of the milk is lower than plasma slightly on acidic side. Basic drugs get trapped in breast milk. Hence can cause foetal adverse effect.

Metochlopramide—loose stool. Opioids—sedation, Antipsychotics—EPS. Co-trimaxozole—neonatal jaundice. Tetracycline—discolouration of teeth.

BIBLIOGRAPHY

1. Katzung DG, Basic and Clinical Pharmacology, Chapter 59, Special Aspect of Perinatal and Paediatric Pharmacology, New York, McGraw-Hill Education Publishing, 2018 (14th edition).

New Drug Delivery System

Drug delivery system is a method or process of drug administration to achieve a therapeutic effect. The drug delivery system is divided into two main types:
- Conventional drug delivery system
- Novel drug delivery system

CONVENTIONAL DRUG DELIVERY SYSTEM

- Classical methods
- Oral
- Buccal/sublingual
- Rectal
- Intravenous
- Subcutaneous
- Intramuscular

Demerits of Conventional Drug Delivery System

- Large amount of drug is delivered to the site
- Therapeutic concentration is not maintained
- Repeated dosage is necessary
- Less patient compliance
- Fluctuations in concentration of drug in blood

NOVEL DRUG DELIVERY SYSTEM (NDDS)

It is a combination of:
- Advance technique/medicinal devices
- New dosage forms

The medication is released at a predetermined site and a predetermined rate over an extended period of time after a single application.

Advantages

- Convenient and patient friendly
- Decreased frequency of administration leads to increased patient compliance
- Controlled rate and slow delivery—sustained therapeutic effect
- Effective concentration for extended time
- Decreased systemic toxicity because it targets a drug specifically to a desired tissue

Various Types of NDDS

Prolonged Release Preparations

Oral

- **Pro-drugs,** e.g. levodopa for Parkinson's disease, sulphasalazine for rheumatoid arthritis and inflammatory bowel disease.
- **Enteric coated tablets and capsules,** e.g. acid resistant coating —prevent gastric irritation—NSAIDs, mesalazine—acrylic polymer release over the length of jejunum, ileum and colon
- Controlled release/extended release/sustained release— drug release in a predetermined manner over extended period of time, e.g. metformin to reduce GIT intolerance, nifedipine—anti-HT (extended therapeutic effect)

Parenteral

For example, insulin (Fig. 26.2)
- Osmotic pumps/portable pumps
- Computerised pumps/implantable pumps
- Pens
- Dermojet
- CSII
  - Patient controlled anaesthesia (PCA), e.g. Fentanyl + propofol
  - Implants/pellets, e.g. norplant (lenonorgesterel implant)
  - Depot preparations, e.g. haloperidol, fluphenazine
- Inhalational drug delivery systems
  - Bronchial asthma—bronchodilators and steroids
    - Metered dose inhaler
    - Dry powder inhalers—rotahalers

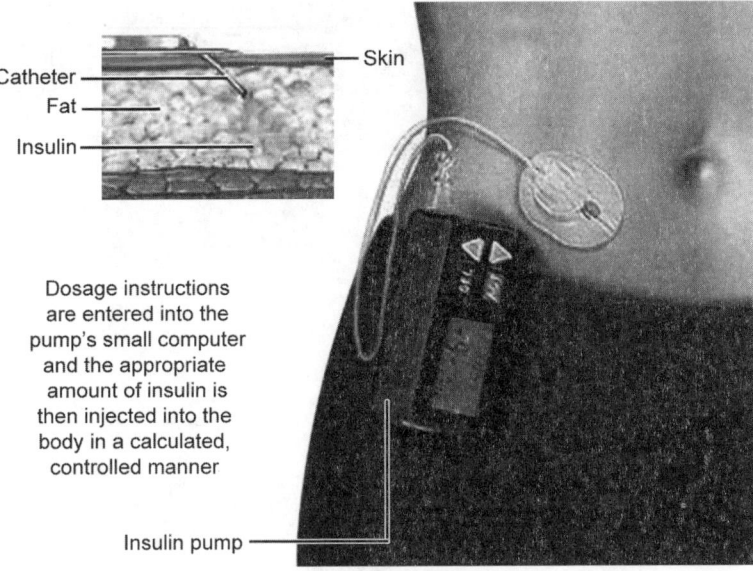

Catheter — Skin
Fat —
Insulin —

Dosage instructions
are entered into the
pump's small computer
and the appropriate
amount of insulin is
then injected into the
body in a calculated,
controlled manner

Insulin pump —

Fig. 26.1: Insulin pump

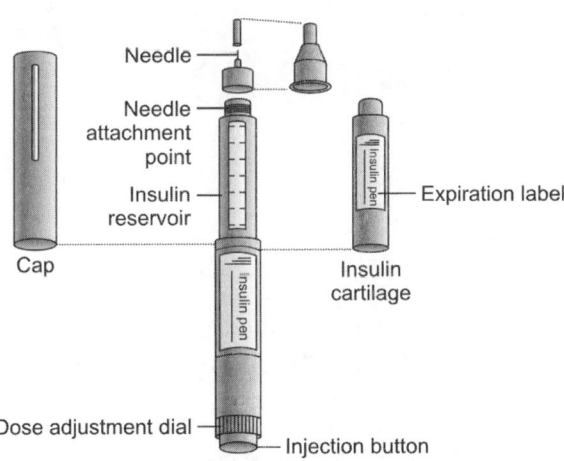

Needle —
Needle
attachment
point
Insulin —
reservoir
Cap
Dose adjustment dial —
Expiration label
Insulin
cartilage
— Injection button

Fig. 26.2: Insulin pen

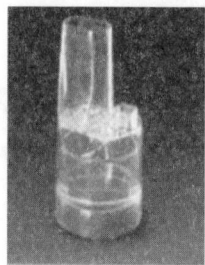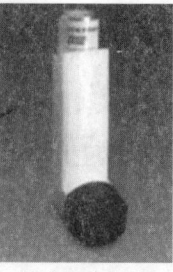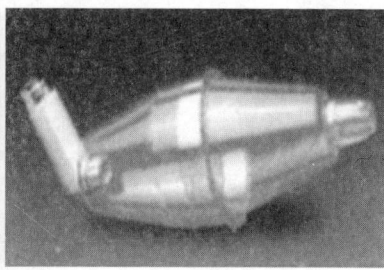

| Rotahaler | Metered dose | Spacer |
| Dry powder inhaler | inhaler or MDI | Space halers |

Fig. 26.3: Inhalation devices

• Inhalational general anaesthetics—vaporizers

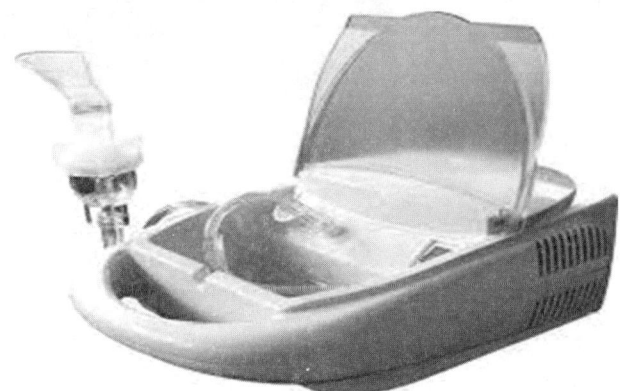

Fig. 26.4: Nebulizer

• Transdermal drug delivery system
  • Devices: Adhesive patches
  • Various shapes and sizes: 5–20 cm^2
  • Deliver the drug at a constant rate
  • Systemic circulation via the stratum corneum
  • Layers
    × Occlusive backing film
    × Rate controlling micropore membrane
    × Drug reservoir
    × Adhesive impregnated with priming dose of the drug.

Advantages

- Maintains constant blood level for longer period without fluctuation.
- Easy to discontinue in case of toxicity
- ↑ patient compliance noninvasive method
- ↓ dose to be administered and ↓ side effects
- ↓ GI effects
- Drug is delivered at a constant and predictable rate
- Irrespective of site of application:
- Usually chest, abdomen, upper arm, lower back, buttock or mastoid region are utilized.
- Examples:
  - *Scopolamine*: Motion sickness (onset 4 hours and duration 72 hours)
  - *Oral dose*: 4–6 hours
  - *Nitroglycerine*: Angina
  - *Clonidine*: Hypertension
  - *Nicotine*: Smokers
  - *Fentanyl*: Pain
  - *Postmenopausal HRT*: Estrogen and progesteron

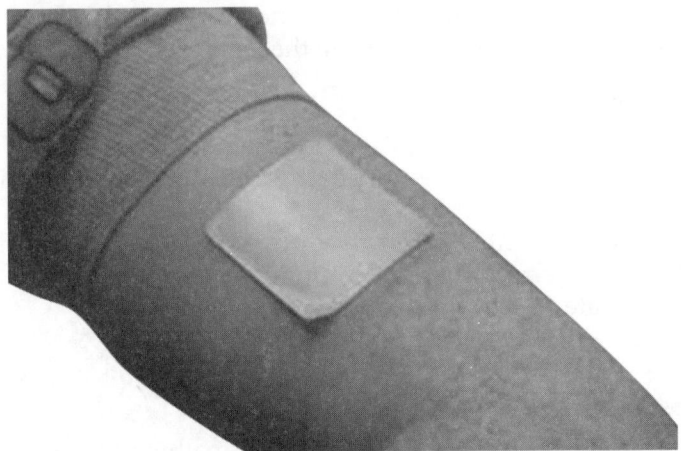

Fig. 26.5: Transdermal patch

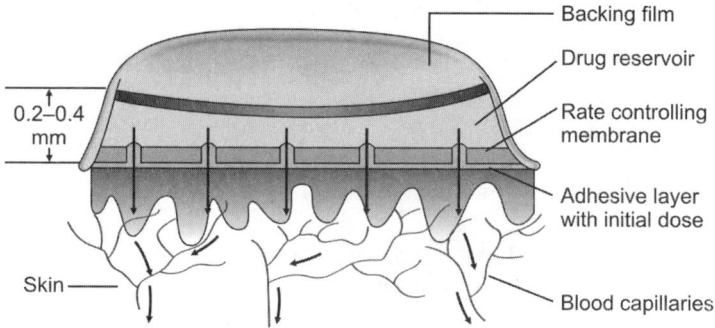

Fig. 26.6: Transdermal patch

LOCAL DELIVERY SYSTEMS

- **Ocusert**
  - ◆ Controlled, delayed and or sustained release bioerodible implantable elements
  - ◆ *Lower conjuctival sac*
  - ◆ Pilocarpineocusert: Glaucoma
  - ◆ 7 days, less side effects and dose also ↓
- Vaginal and uterine systems
  - ◆ *Progestasert*: IUCD (60 µg/d of progesterone for 1 year)
  - ◆ Dinoprostone vaginal insert for cervical ripening—labour
- Iontophoresis
  Mild electric current applied for the transport of drug across the skin, e.g. vasopressin, dexamethasone

Drug Eluting Stents (DES)

It is done to avoid restenosis in post-angioplasty patients. The lumen of the stents are embedded with drugs embedded in a surface polymer.

Examples: Antiproliferative agents like tacrolimus, everolimus, sirolimus, leflunomide, methyprednisolone, methotrexate, vincristine.

TARGETED DELIVERY SYSTEMS

Liposomes

They are bilayered vesicles made of amphipathic phospholipids, e.g. liposomal amphotericin B

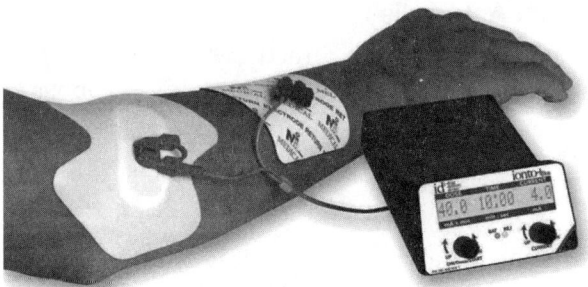

Fig. 26.7: Iontophoresis

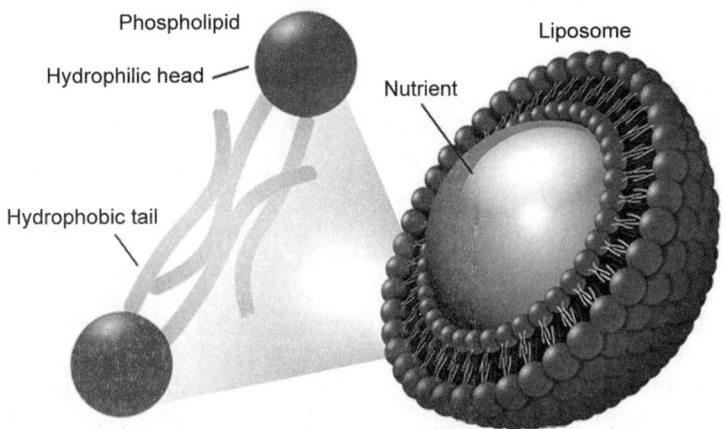

Fig. 26.8: Design of a liposome

Nanoparticles

It is the science of manipulating matter at nanoscale. The drug is conjugated with a nanoparticle. It is easily penetrated in different tissues in a specific target. They are made up of biological materials like albumin, gelatin and phospholipids or synthetic polymers. Depending on the shape they can be of many types like nanospheres, nanotubes, miscelle, dendrimers,

Examples: Paclitaxel, doxorubicin, tissue plasminogen activator, tamoxifene

Monoclonal Antibodies

Monoclonal antibodies act directly when binding to a cancer specific antigen and induce immunological response to cancer cells.

Antibodies: Target the antigens specifically.

So less adverse effects

Examples:

- Infliximab, adalimumab (inhibits TNF-α)—rheumatoid arthritis, Crohn's disease, ulcerative
- Basiliximab, daclizumab (inhibits IL-2 on activated T cells)—used in acute rejection of kidney transplant
- Omalizumab (anti-IgE)—moderate-to-severe allergic asthma.

Gene Therapy

It is the field of biotechnology which deals with introduction of functional genetic material into the target cells. This may be done for multiple reasons:

- Replace or supplement defective genes.
- To modify target cells.
- To achieve therapeutic goals.

The two methods which are employed for gene therapy are:

- Gene modification.
- Gene transfer: Physical, chemical or biological delivery methods.

Uses

- Genetically linked diseases, e.g. cystic fibrosis, growth hormone deficiency, Duchenne's muscular dystrophy, sickle cell anaemia.
- Cancers.
- Neurodegenerative diseases, e.g. Alzheimer's disease, multiple sclerosis, stroke.

BIBLIOGRAPHY

1. Tiwari G et al, Drug delivery system; an updated review, International Journal of Pharmaceuticals Investigations, Jan 2012, Vol 2, Issue 1, 1–11.

Chronopharmacology

It is a branch of pharmacology that deals with the variations in the pharmacological response of various drugs in relation with biological timings and endogenous periodicity.

Various types of biological rhythms are shown in Fig. 27.1.

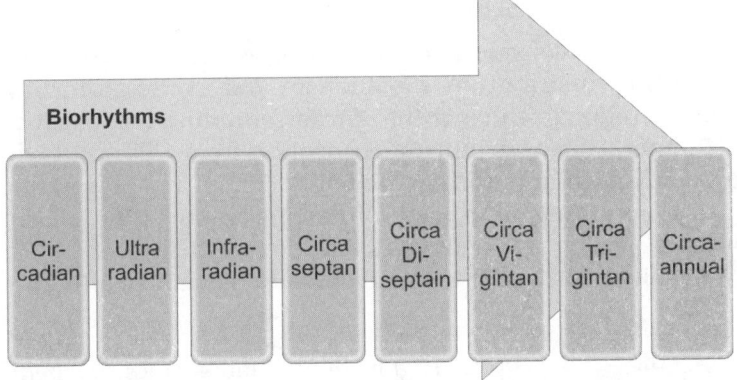

Biorhythms							
Cir-cadian	Ultra radian	Infra-radian	Circa septan	Circa Di-septain	Circa Vi-gintan	Circa Tri-gintan	Circa-annual
T < 24 h	T ~ 24 h	T < 24 h	T = 7 d	T = 14 d	T = 21 d	T = 30 d	T = 1 y

Fig. 27.1: Different rhythms in our body

Examples
• Ultradian—90 min REM cycle
• Circadian—hormone release, platelet aggregation, HMG CoA reductase activity, blood cortisol levels .
• Infradian—menstruation
• Circaseptan—work rest scheme

- Circa-annual—1 year—migration of birds, seasonal mood changes

BRANCHES

Various branches of chronobiology are chronophysiology, chronopathology and chronopharmacology.

Chronopharmacology further deals with chronotherapeutics, chronokinetic, chronodynamics and chronotoxicity.

Chronotherapeutics

It deals with the application of principles of chronobiology in the treatment of diseases.

It deals with the increase of the efficiency and safety of the drug by providing its concentrations in relation with the 24 hours in synchrony with biological rhythm determinants of disease.

Chronopharmacokinetics

This takes into consideration of pharmacokinetic processes like absorption, distribution, metabolism and excretion for time administration to enhance the efficacy or reduce the toxicity.

Temporal changes in drug absorption from GIT occurs due to circadian variations in gastric acid secretion and pH, motility, gastric emptying time, gastrointestinal blood flow, plasma protein binding and drug distribution and drug metabolism. Lipid soluble drugs are better absorbed when given after food.

Kinetic processes	Application
Absorption Nifedipine, nitrates and propranolol	• Highly lipid soluble drugs are better absorbed in the morning. • Skin penetration of LA is better in the evening
Distribution Antiepileptic drugs, diazepam, prednisolone	• Free drug concentration is high in the night. • Plasma proteins—reduced in the evening
Metabolism Phenobarbital, cyclophosphamide	• Hepatic blood flow—high in the morning. • Enzyme activity higher in the evening
Elimination	• GFR, renal blood flow, urinary pH, tubular reabsorption • Higher value in daytime

Chronopharmacodynamics

This deals with the study of variation in the pharmacological response in relation with the biological rhythm at cellular and subcellular level. Various parameters which affect this response are variation in the number of receptors, second messengers, metabolic pathways, sympathetic and parasympathetic activities, e.g. cell cycle and noncell cycle specific anticancer drugs. Examples:

1. Statins
2. Anticancer drugs and cell cycle specificity
3. Ace inhibitors
4. Anti-inflammatory

Chronotoxicity

This deals with the study of relation between drug toxicity and biological variations in physiological process. Example: Administration of long-acting methyl prednisolone, toxicity can be reduced by giving in morning time.

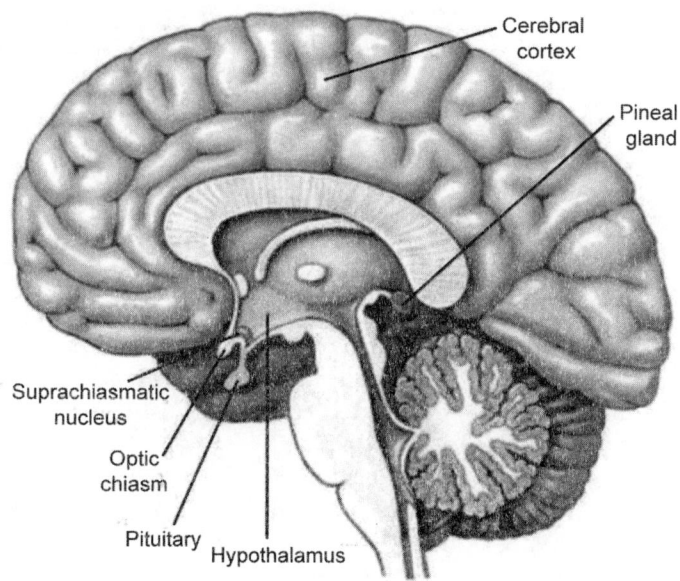

Fig. 27.2: CNS site controlling circadian rhythm

Mechanisms explaining Chronopharmacology

Suprachiasmatic nucleus (master clock) in the hypothalamus and pineal gland control the biological clock in the body through retino-hypothalamic tract which get affected by light signals. Pineal gland plays its part by release of melatonin (sleep hormone). Circadian rhythms are also reflected by various physiological processes like feeding, sleep-wakefulness, hormone secretion, metabolic homeostasis and autonomic processes.

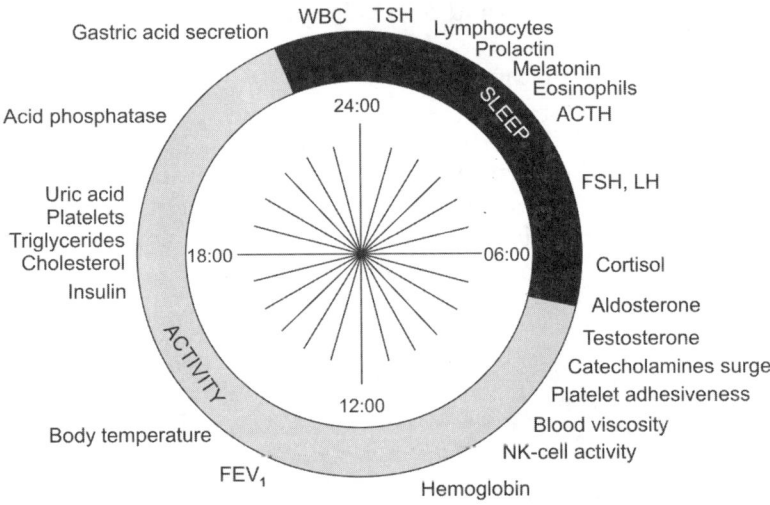

Fig. 27.3: Physiological functions showing circadian rhythm

Therapeutic applications in relation with the chronopharmacology:

1. **Cardiovascular events:** Acute myocardial infarction, sudden cardiac death, angina pectoris, transient ischemic attacks/stroke—high incidence of these episodes are between 6 am and 12 noon.

   Rationale: Increased vascular tone, increased platelet aggregation, and decreased intrinsic thrombolytic activity during this period.

   Control onset extended release (COER) verapamil: Mechanism—shell dissolves slowly. Taken at bedtime, peak effect from 5 am to 12 noon. No midnight drop in blood pressure.

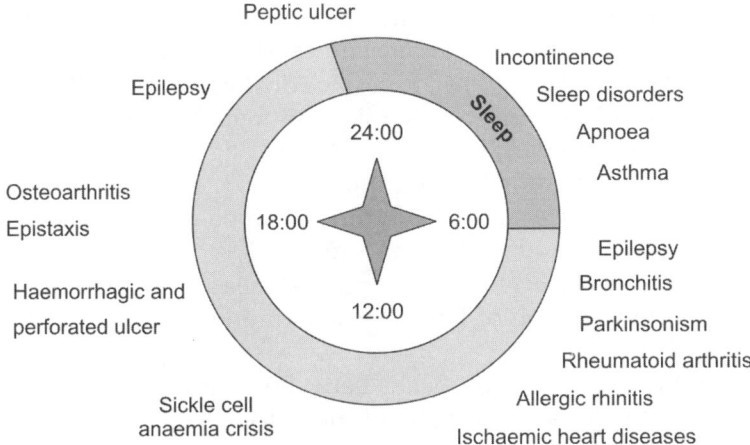

Fig. 27.4: Diseases in relation with the circadian rhythm

- *ACE inhibitors*: At bedtime for better control of BP.
- *Aspirin:* To be given at bedtime to have maximum anti-platelet effect in the morning.
- *Statins:* To be given in the evening as HMG-COA activity is higher in the evening.

2. **Bronchial asthma:** Acute attack of asthma is more common in early morning between 4 am and 6 am.
   - *Rationale*: Increased bronchoconstriction at night due to →↑parasympathetic tone, ↓adrenaline, decreased cortisol at midnight, increased sensitivity to irritants and allergens at night—higher concentration of IgE and histamine.
   - Theophylline and beta 2 agonist is timed at evening—to have higher effect.

3. **Endocrine system:** Highest secretion of cortisol early morning and lowest at midnight, GH peaks during sleep, testosterone peaks early morning. TSH peaks at midnight. Application:
   - Corticosteroids given as single morning dose cause less pituitary adrenal suppression
   - Inhaled corticosteroid in bronchial asthma—single dose at 5.00 pm
   - Early morning hyperglycemia is seen in the Type-2 DM.

- *Dawn phenomenon:* Early morning rise in the corticos-teroid, growth hormone and catecholamine.
- *Somogy phenomenon:* Excessive dose of insulin will cause midnight hypoglycaemia. This will lead to compensatory hyperglycaemia or overeating causing increase blood sugar in the morning.
- *ADH analogues*: At bedtime to avoid bed wetting in children and nocturia in adults.
- *OC pills*: Development of phased pills and depends upon the variation of female sex hormone in the menstrual cycle.

4. **GIT:** Acid secretion peaks between 10 pm and 2 am and ulcer pain is worst at this time. Ulcer healing is directly related to acid secretion.
   - *Application*: Evening dosage of H2 receptor antagonists or PPI are highly effective.

5. **CNS-Melatonin:** Secreted at night by pineal gland which induces sleep.
   - *Application:* Bedtime administration of sedative hypnotics will be more effective, e.g. melatonin agonist—ramelteon.

6. **Musculoskeletal system**
   - *Rheumatoid arthritis:* Symptoms more severe—8 am and 11 am.
   - *Application:* Long acting NSAIDs at bedtime will be more effective.

   Osteoarthritis: Pain more intense between 2 pm and 8 pm.
   - *Application:* Morning dose for afternoon worsening, evening dose for nighttime worsening.

   Hypercholesterolemia

7. **Hyperlipidemia:** Cholesterol synthesis more at night.
   - Evening dose of HMG-CoA reductase inhibitors is more effective.

8. **Cancer:** Cancer cells are considered to have lost internal time keeping mechanism.
   - *Application:* Tumour cells and normal cells differ in their chronobiological cycles. The basis for the chrono-pharmacotherapy of cancers.

Lymphoma

- The DNA synthesis in the normal human bone marrow cells has a peak around noon while the peak of DNA synthesis in lymphoma cells is around midnight.
- So, an s-phase active cytotoxic therapy at late nights should be more advantageous.

9. **Skin disorders**
   - *Psoriasis*: Cell proliferation rate peaks between 9 pm and 3 am and inflammatory activity highest at night, least in the morning.
   - *Atopic dermatitis*: Sensitivity to histamine highest at night.
   - *Topical corticosteroids*: Activity in the afternoon higher than that in the morning.

CONCLUSION

Effectiveness and toxicity of a drug are not constant over 24-hr period.

Understanding the biological rhythms can optimize and individualize drug therapy to a great extent.

Thus it can help to decrease the drug related toxicity and enhance effectiveness.

CHRONOPHARMACEUTICAL TECHNOLOGIES

Parenteral routes
- Chronomodulating infusion pumps
- Controlled-release microchips

Oral Routes

Given below are examples of chronopharmaceutical technologies e.g. CODOS, chronotherapeutic oral drug absorption system (CODAS), OROS, CEFORM TIMERx, polymers, microchips, diffucaps

Principle

This method involves physicochemical modification of the active ingredient and/or the use of controlled-release erodible polymer.

Pulsatile Drug Delivery Systems

Here a targeted drug is delivered at specific site due to induction of certain physiochemical stimuli at target site.

This technology is useful for the disease condition like bronchial asthma, angina pectoris and rheumatoid arthritis.

CODOS	*Multi-particulate pH dependent system*	*Verapamil*	*Hypertension*
DIFFUCAPS	Multi-particulate system	Verapamil and propranolol	Hypertension
OROS	Osmotic mechanism	Verapamil	Hypertension
PULSINCAP	Rupturable system	Dofetilide	Hypertension

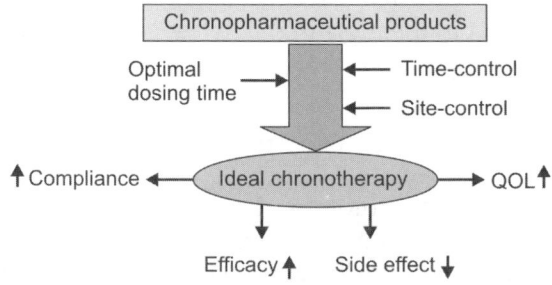

Fig. 27.5: Ideal chronotherapy

BIBLIOGRAPHY

1. Laxminarayana K Bairy, Chronotherapeutics: A hype or future of chronopharmacology? 2013, 45(6); 545–546, Indian Journal of Pharmacology.
2. Sagar Singh Jough et al, Chronopharmacology: Recent advancements in the treatment of Diabetes Mellitus through Chronotherapy, Human Journals Review Article, May 2017, 9(2).

Drug Transporters

Membrane proteins that control the influx of essential nutrients and ions and the efflux of cellular waste, environmental toxins and other xenobiotics.

Two major superfamily of transporters—
- ATP binding cassettes (ABC) and
- Solute carrier (SLC) transporter

ATP binding cassettes (ABC)	Solute carriers (SLC)
• Primary active transporters mediate unidirectional efflux	• Secondary active and facilitated transporters mediate both drug uptake and efflux
• P-glycoprotein (P-gp or MDR1)	• Organic cation transporters (OCTs)
• Multidrug resistance associated protein 2 (MRP 2)	• Organic anion transporters (OATs)
• Breast cancer resistance protein (BCRP)	• Organic anion transporting polypeptides (OATPs)
• *Examples:* Anticancer drugs, protease inhibitors, hormones, digoxin	• Examples: Metformin, diuretics, antidepressants

Important Properties
- Bind to substrates, changes conformation, and release them on the other side of the membrane
- Specific, saturable, inhibitable
- Structure:
  - *Transmembrane domains (TMDs):* Substrate-binding site—responsible for substrate specificity.

- *Nucleotide-binding domain (NBD):* ATP binding site.
- Vectorial transport: Asymmetrical transport across a monolayer of polarized cells.
- Examples:
  - Absorption of nutrients, bile acids, drugs from intestine.
  - Hepatic and urinary excretion of drugs from blood to lumen.
  - Efflux of drugs from brain's endothelial and epithelial cells.

ROLE OF TRANSPORTERS

Pharmacokinetics

- **Absorption:** Selective uptake and efflux of drugs, e.g. PEPT-1 helps in absorption of lactam antibiotics, ACE inhibitors.
- **Distribution:** Mediate entry or efflux of drugs in different cells, e.g. P-gp efflux anticancer drugs from blood–brain barrier.
- **Metabolism:** By controlling drug's access to the enzymes, e.g. statins, ARBs, irinotecan, fexofenadine are some of the substrates of OATP1B1 and MRP2 transporters in liver.
- **Excretion:** Elimination of drugs by hepatic and renal routes, e.g. P-gp actively secretes digoxin, tacrolimus, BCRP efflux topotecan from GIT and placenta.

Pharmacodynamics

They have a role in processes which control effect of drug:
- Delivery to site of action, e.g. anticancer drugs are effluxed in brain
- Control of tissue concentrations
- **Act as drug targets:** GABA transporters (GAT)—target for tiagabine, valproate, norepinephrine transporters (NET)—target for TCA and cocaine.
- **Drug interactions**, e.g. probenecid reduce irinotecan induced diarrhea, digoxin concentration increased by quinidine.
- **Drug resistance:** P-glycoprotein, BCRP, MRPs are efflux transporter associated with resistance to cytotoxic anticancer drugs, antiviral drugs.
- **Adverse drug reactions,** e.g. increased concentration of digoxin, cyclosporin in brain is due to reduced P-gp efflux,

metformin-induced lactic acidosis due to increased uptake by OCT1 in liver.

- Polymorphism in transporter genes play a crucial role in clinical drug response, e.g. OATP1B1 associated with statin-induced myopathy, SLC22A with metformin. Examples:
  - **Neurotransmitter transporters** for drugs used in neuropsychiatric disorders. Examples:
    - *GABA transporters (GAT):* Target for tiagabine, valproate.
    - *Norepinephrine transporters (NET):* Target for TCA and cocaine
    - *Dopamine transporters (DAT):* Target for cocaine, amphetamine.
    - *Serotonin transporters (SERT):* Target for SSRIs and TCAs.
  - **Cholesterol transporters**—cardiovascular disease, e.g. NPC1L1.
  - **Glucose transporters** in metabolic syndrome, e.g. SGLT 2 in diabetes mellitus.
  - **Na$^+$–K$^+$ antiporters** in hypertension, e.g. loop and thiazide diuretics.

P-gp/MDR1

- Most important ABC transporter.
- Permeability glycoprotein (P-gp), multidrug resistance protein 1 (MDR1).
- Encoded by the ABCB1 gene.
- Extensively distributed and expressed in the intestine, liver, kidney, capillary endothelial cells in the blood–brain and blood–testis barrier.
- It is an efflux pump with wide substrate specificity
- Increased intestinal expression can reduce the absorption of drugs.
- Plays important role in anticancer drug resistance.

Examples of P-gp Substrates

- *Anticancer:* Vincristine, vinblastine, doxorubicin, dauno-rubicin, paclitaxel
- *Protease inhibitors:* Indinavir, ritunavir
- *Immunosuppressants:* Tacrolimus, cyclosporine, dexamethasone
- *Cardiac:* Quinidine, digoxin

- *Anticonvulsants:* Carbamazepine, phenytoin
- *Others*: Atorvastatin, terfenadine, ondansetron, erythromycin

P-gp Inhibitors

Inhibition of P-gp represents a promising approach for treatmenting multidrug-resistant tumours.

Examples of P-gp Inhibitors

- Verapamil
- Quinidine
- Vaspodar
- Elacidar

BIBLIOGRAPHY

1. Goodman and Gilman's The Pharmacological Basis of Therapeutics, 12th Edition, The McGraw-Hill Companies, Chapter 5, Cathleen M.Giacomimi, yuichisugiyamma.

29

Ion Channels

Ion channels are transmembrane proteins that create a gated, water-filled pore to allow flow of ions between the intracellular and the extracellular environments.

Important Characteristics

- Highly selective in type of ion transported (exceptions are there).
- Very high rate of ion transfer.
- Ions are transported across electrochemical gradient.
- Passive mechanism

Physiological Roles

- Maintaining resting membrane potential
- Nerve impulse conduction
- Generation of action potential, synaptic transmission.
- Cardiac, skeletal and smooth muscle contraction.
- Epithelial transport of nutrients and ions.
- T-cell activation (immune regulation).
- Pancreatic beta cell insulin release.

Ion channels are classified into two main types:

Voltage gated: The stimulus is change in membrane potential, e.g. sodium, potassium, calcium.

Ligand gated: The stimulus is binding of a ligand/substrate to the ion channel, e.g. acetylcholine, serotonin, glycine.

Other stimuli: In response to chemical stimuli, temperature changes or mechanical force.

Parts of an Ion Channel

- Different subunits
- Gates which open and close in response to specific stimulus
- Pore—passage which allows flow of ions through the channel
- Ion selectivity filter—regulates which ions are permitted through the pore

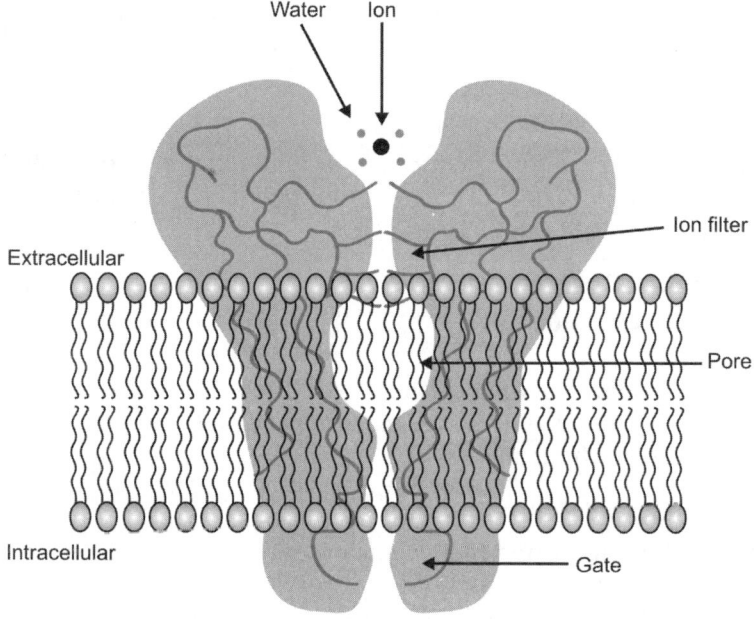

Examples of diseases which are related with abnormality in ion channels are given in Table 29.1.

TABLE 29.1: Diseases related with abnormality in ion channels

Ion channel	Type	Diseases
Potassium channel	Kir	Bartter's syndrome, neonatal diabetes
Potassium channel	Kv	Sur2-dilated cardiomyopathy KCNQ1/hERG—long QT syndrome
Sodium channel	Na	Epilepsy, cerebellar ataxia
Transient receptor potential channel	TRP	Polycystic kidney disease, familial episodic pain syndrome

TABLE 29.2: Drugs and ion channel

Drugs	Ion channel	Indication
Diltiazem, verapamil, nifedipine	L-type calcium channels	hypertension
lamotrigine	Voltage gated sodium channels	Epilepsy, bipolar disorder
Lidocaine, bupivacaine	Voltage gated sodium channels	Local anaesthetics
Gabapentin, pregabalin	Voltage gated calcium channels	Neuropathic pain
Varenicline	Nicotinic acetylcholine receptor	Smoking cessation
Flupirtine, retigabine	KCNQ potassium channels	Epilepsy
Sotalol	hERG potassium channels	Arrhythmia
Flecainide	Voltage gated sodium channels	Arrhythmia
Phenytoin, lacosamide, carbamazepine	Voltage gated sodium channels	Epilepsy
Riluzole	Voltage gated sodium channels	Amyotrophic lateral sclerosis

Potassium Channels

- Important for maintaining electrical gradient across cell membrane
- Important role in several physiological processes
  - Insulin release
  - Electrical activity in heart
  - Pain signaling
  - Signal transmission in nerves and muscle

They are bidirectional so flow of ions can be in any direction. The flow of ions is usually from intracellular to extracellular compartment, that is efflux of potassium ions.

Types of K^+ channels depending on number of transmembrane (TM) domains:

TABLE 29.3: Types of K⁺ channels depending on number of transmembrane (TM) domains

Number of TM domains	Name of channel	Examples
2TM Family	Inward rectifier (Kir)	ATP sensitive potassium channels in heart and pancreatic cells
4TM Family	Two-pore K⁺ channels (K2P)	Mechano-gated K⁺ channels
6TM Family	Voltage-gated K⁺ channels (Kv)	Neurons (epilepsy)
	Small conductance (SK)	Ca²⁺ activated K⁺ channels
	Slo channel	BKCa channels have role in cerebral ischaemia

Depending on the action of drugs on potassium channels, they are classified as:
- **K⁺ channel openers:** Used as vasodilators, anti-hypertensive.
- **K⁺ channel blockers:** Used as anti-diabetic, anti-arrhythmic.

TABLE 29.4: Current and proposed use of K⁺ channel openers

K⁺ channel openers	Current use in the therapy	Newer proposed use
1. Nicorandil	Vasodilators and antihypertensive	Erectile dysfunction
2. Minoxidil	Angina	Premature labour
3. Pinnacidil	CHF	PVD (Reynold's disease)
4. Diazoxide	Alopecia	Urinary incontinence
5. Chromakalin	Insulinoma	Bronchial asthma
Class III		
Antiarrhythmic	**Antiarrhythmic**	
1. Vernacalent		
2. Bretyllium		
3. Dofetilide		
4. Azimilide		
5. Tedisamil		
6. Sotalol		

Contd.

TABLE 29.4: Current and proposed use of K⁺ channel openers (*Contd.*)

K⁺ channel openers	Current use in the therapy	Newer proposed use
Sufonylurea		
• Tolbutamide and others	Antidiabetic	
Na⁺ channel blocker		
Anti-epileptics		
• Phenytoin Na		
• Valproic acid		
• Carbamazepine		
• Lamotrigine		
• Topiramate		
• Zonisamide		
Local anaesthetics		
Antiarrhythmics		
Class I (A, B, C)		
• Quinidine		
• Procainamide		
• Propafenone		
• Flecainide		
Few toxins		
• Tetrodo-toxin		
Present in the fish		
• Saxi-toxin		
Calcium channel blocker	Three types	
	Voltage sensitive	
	L-type: Heart and vascular smooth muscle	
	• DHPs and Non-DHPs	
	Example: Nifedipine, diltiazem, verapamil	
	T-type: Neurones	
	• Ethosuccimide	
	• Flunnarazine	

Contd.

TABLE 29.4: Current and proposed use of K⁺ channel openers (*Contd.*)

K^+ channel openers	Current use in the therapy	Newer proposed use
	N-type: Neurones	
	• Pregabaline	
	• Gabapentine	
	Receptor operated	
	Leak channel	
Ligand gated ion channels	• Barbiturates	Major ligand in the CNS are
	• Benzodiazepine	
Cl channel opener (GABA mimetics)	• Opioids	1. Acetylcholine-linked Na channel
	• General anaesthetics	
	• Alcohols	2. Glutamate-linked ion channels
	• Lubiprostone (IBD)	3. 5 HT3-linked ion channels

BIBLIOGRAPHY

1. Bagal S et al, Ion channels as therapeutic targets: A drug discovery perspective, J.Med. Chem. 2013;56;593–624.

Phosphodiesterase (PDE) Inhibitors

Phosphodiesterase (PDE) is involved in metabolism of camp. Inhibitors of PDE are associated with increased camp and phosphorylation of protein kinase which further leads to increased Ca$^+$.

There are five different isoforms of phosphodiesterase (PDE).

TABLE 30.1: Types of PDE inhibitors

Type of PDE inhibitors	Drugs	Special properties and uses
Non-selective PDE inhibitors	• Aminiphyllin, theophylline • Pentoxy-phylline • Caffeine	• Used in bronchial asthma • Peripheral vascular disease, neuro-pathic pain • CNS stimulant
PDE 1 inhibitors	• Vinpocetine (vinca alkaloid) • Nicardipine • Nimodipine	• Increased cerebral blood flow/ neuroprotective: Dementia • Coronary selective, less myocardial depression • Cross BBB, cerebral blood vessels selective: Migraine, cerebral stroke (decreased mortality)
PDE 2 inhibitors	• Oxindole (tryptophan derivative)	• Levels increase in hepatic ence-phalopathy, sepsis and respiratory distress. • Anti HIV, anti-cancer, anti-hyper-tensive, anti-convulsant properties

Contd.

TABLE 30.1: Types of PDE inhibitors *(Contd.)*

Type of PDE inhibitors	Drugs	Special properties and uses
PDE 3 inhibitors	• Cilastazole • Amrinone/ milrinine • Anagrelide	• Peripheral vascular disease, anti-platelet • Ionodilators used in CHF • Chronic myeloid leukemia
PDE 4 inhibitors	• Roflumilast • Drotaverine	• COPD/asthma • Anti-spasmodic
PDE 5 inhibitors	• Sildenafil, vardanafil, tadalafil • Dipyridamole	• Erectile dysfunction, pulmonary hypertension (blue vision—PDE 6 inhibition effect) • Angina, antiplatelet (ADR—coronary steel phenomenon)
PDE 10 inhibitors	• Papaverine	• Role in psychosis

BIBLIOGRAPHY

1. Ghosh R et al. Phosphoditerase inhibitors: Their role and implication. International journal of PharmaTech Research Oct 2009, Vol.1(4): 1148–60.

Stem Cell Therapy

Stem cells are cells found in all multicellular organisms that can multiply and differentiate into various specialized cell types. They can also self-renew to produce more stem cells. So the essential properties of all stem cells are:
- **Self-renewal:** Ability to multiply through mitotic division.
- **Differentiation:** Capacity to differentiate into specialized cells.

Differentiation

It is the process where unspecialized cells give rise to specialized mature cells in response to different internal and external stimulus.
- Internal stimulus, e.g. genes
- External stimulus, e.g. chemicals like growth factors, cytokines.

Depending on their ability to differentiate they are classified into the following types:
- **Totipotent:** Can differentiate into embryonic and extra-embryonic cell types, e.g. morula stage.
- **Pluripotent:** Can differentiate into nearly all cell types, e.g. cells in blastocyst.
- **Multipotent:** Can differentiate into cells of a closely related family, e.g. haematopoetic cells.
- **Oligopotent:** Can differentiate into only a few cells. e.g. lymphoid cells.

- **Unipotent:** Can divide into only one cell type, e.g. muscle cells, cardiac cells.

  Main types of stem cells are:
  - *Embryonic stem cells:* Isolated from the inner cell mass of blastocyst.
  - *Fetal stem cells:* Isolated from foetal tissue at later stages.
  - Amniotic stem cells.
  - Umbilical cord stem cells.
  - *Adult stem cells:* Found in various tissues.
  - *Others:* Induced pleuripotent stem cells, somatic cell nuclear transfer.

EMBRYONIC STEM CELLS

They are pleuripotent cells derived from inner cell mass of the blastocyst (5–6 days of intrauterine life). The sources were the embryos produced by *in vitro* fertilization for infertility treatment.

Steps in the synthesis of embryonic stem cells:
- Embryos are collected and cryopreserved.
- Thawed and cultured to blastocyst stage.
- Cells from inner cell mass are isolated.
- Cultured on embryonic feeder cell layer in the presence of fibroblast growth factor (FGF–2), sox4, oct2 which promotes cell multiplication but prevent differentiation.
- Depending on what type of specialized cells are needed, they are provided respective growth factors, e.g. cardiac cells, skin cells.

FOETAL STEM CELLS

- Usually derived from aborted foetal tissue
- Limited renewal capacity

AMNIOTIC FLUID DERIVED STEM CELLS

- Multipotent
- Very active and can multiply rapidly
- Can differentiate in cells of adipogenic, osteogenic, myogenic, endothelial, hepatic and also neuronal lines.
- It can be used for autologous transplant as well as on others.

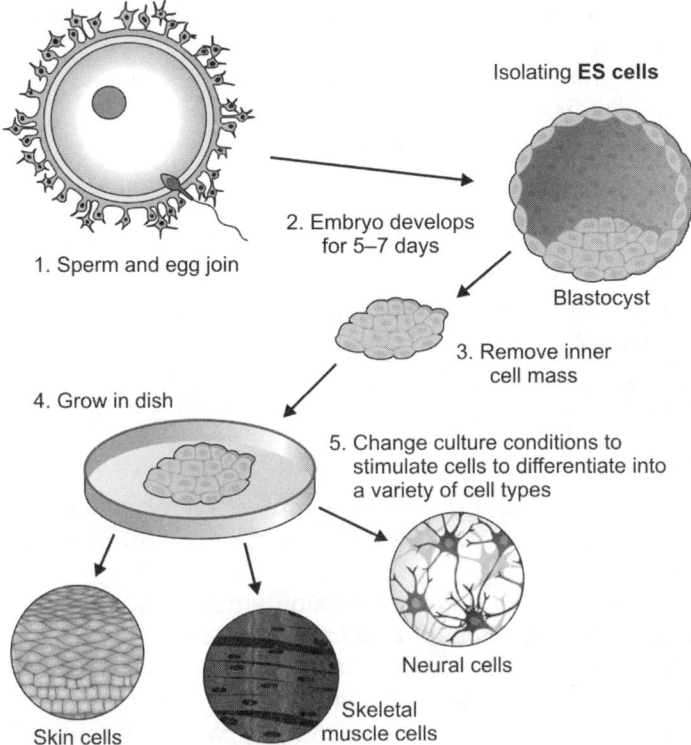

Isolating **ES cells**

2. Embryo develops
for 5–7 days

1. Sperm and egg join

Blastocyst

3. Remove inner
cell mass

4. Grow in dish

5. Change culture conditions to
stimulate cells to differentiate into
a variety of cell types

Neural cells

Skeletal
muscle cells

Skin cells

Fig. 31.1: Steps in the synthesis of embryonic stem cells

UMBILICAL CORD STEM CELLS

- Cells are taken from umbilical cord blood just after birth.
- This involves the least risk because they are patients own cells called autologous cells .
- They are stored so that they may be used later if the subject develops disease.
- They can be differentiated into the required cell types.
- For example, neural cells for Parkinson's disease, blood cells for leukemia cases

ADULT STEM CELLS/SOMATIC CELLS

There are a group of stem cells normally present in our body to replace the dead and damaged cells, e.g. hematopoetic cells, epithelial cells in skin, hair, gut.

The advantages of adult stem cells over foetal/embryonic cells are:
- Less chances of immune reaction and rejection.
- Less ethical issues.
- Less likely to form tumours.

Disadvantages
- Less number of cells, so difficult to isolate.
- Limited differentiation.

The accessible sources of stem cells in adult are:
- Bone marrow
- Adipose tissue
- Blood

USES
- Drug discovery and development—screening of potential drugs, e.g. cancer cell lines for anticancer agents are already used for screening.
- Toxicity studies—rather than using whole animals, potential drugs can be screened for toxicity in cell lines.
- Cell-based therapy (regenerative medicine), e.g. multiple sclerosis, stroke, spinal cord injury, cartilage cells in osteoarthritis, carcinomas, leukemias, pancreatic islet cells in diabetes
- Gene therapy

IMPORTANT CONCERNS
- Stem cell development or proliferation must be controlled once placed into patients.
- High risk of rejection of stem cell transplants
- Risk of contamination by viruses, bacteria, fungi and mycoplasma is possible.
- Ethical issues (guidelines for stem cell research were published by ICMR in 2013).

BIBLIOGRAPHY

1. Larijani B. et al, Stem cell therapy in treatment of different diseases, Acta Medica Iranica, Feb 2012, Vol 50, issue 2; 79–96.

Index